# The Medical Evaluation of Psychiatric Patients

# The Medical Evaluation of Psychiatric Patients

**Randolph B. Schiffer, M.D., and**
**Robert F. Klein, M.D.**
*The University of Rochester School of Medicine and Dentistry*
*Rochester, New York*

**and**

**Roger C. Sider, M.D.**
*Pine Rest Christian Hospital*
*Grand Rapids, Michigan*

SPRINGER SCIENCE+BUSINESS MEDIA, LLC

Library of Congress Cataloging in Publication Data

Schiffer, Randolph B.
The medical evaluation of psychiatric patients / Randolph B. Schiffer, Robert F. Klein, and Roger C. Sider.
p. cm.
Includes bibliographies and index.
ISBN 978-1-4899-0785-1 ISBN 978-1-4899-0783-7 (eBook)
DOI 10.1007/978-1-4899-0783-7
1. Mentally ill—Medical examinations. 2. Neurologic examination. I. Klein, Robert F. (Robert Frederick), 1929- . II. Sider, Roger C. III. Title.
[DNLM: 1. Mental Disorders. 2. Neurologic Examination. 3. Physical Examination. WM 100 S333m]
RC469.S33 1988
616.89'075—dc19
DNLM/DLC 88-25380
for Library of Congress CIP


Originally published by Plenum Publishing Corporation New York in 1988
Softcover reprint of the hardcover 1st edition 1988

Dedicated to

Brenton

and his mother, Lynn;

Connie;

and Joann

# Foreword

One of the fascinations of psychiatry is that it is amenable to many different approaches. In seeking to account for mental disorder, for example, it is possible to explore the meaning and significance of symptoms in the psychodynamic sense, to examine the social determinants of illness, or to adopt an essentially biological viewpoint in investigating links between physiological and psychological dysfunction. As a clinical discipline it may be practiced in the community, in the specialized clinic or hospital, or shoulder-to-shoulder with other medical practitioners in the general hospital. This richness and diversity are at once a strength and a weakness, attracting practitioners with a wide range of talents and interests, yet sometimes leading to polarizations and false antitheses.

The so-called "medical model" of psychiatry has come under a good deal of attack, and deservedly so when claiming an exclusive provenance over all types and aspects of mental disorder. What cannot be gainsaid, however, is the central role of medicine in relation to many parts of the field, and the success in terms of understanding and therapy that has resulted from medicine's involvement. Nor can it be doubted, after the most cursory acquaintance with the physically or mentally ill, that the relationship between these two forms of suffering is often so close and so mutually reinforcing that distinctions are drawn somewhat arbitrarily. This last is perhaps the cardinal reason for the alliance between medicine and psychiatry.

The present book can be viewed as a painstaking illustration of this very theme. The approach of Dr. Schiffer and his colleagues is avowedly medical in displaying links between somatic and psychic dysfunction. Indeed, it is rather the reverse, in that they start each time with the psychiatric disorder and proceed from there to discuss possible physical pathologies that may provoke, augment, or release it. This has the advantage that we are alerted throughout to a range of somatic disorders that may all too easily come to be overlooked in the psychiatric patient yet which can be crucially relevant to the genesis of his problems.

In all parts of the book the authors maintain a soundly clinical stance, the essence of which is that we must remain cognizant of those patterns that recur and of connections that are made most frequently. They draw on wide experience at the interface between internal medicine and neurology on the one hand and psychiatry on the other to stress what are the *likely* somatic concomitants of different forms of mental disorder. In this way we are spared reliance on exhaustive and exhausting lists. We find instead a readable and useful text that should be widely successful in encouraging psychiatrists to appraise their patients thoroughly in the physical domain. If this aim is achieved, vast numbers of patients will undoubtedly be benefited.

W. A. Lishman
*Institute of Psychiatry*
*De Crespigny Park*
*Denmark Hill*
*London, England*

# Preface

Our purpose in writing this book has been to provide mental health clinicians with practical guidance for the medical evaluation of their patients. We have especially considered the diagnostic issues faced by practicing psychiatrists in its preparation, but we hope it may prove of interest as well to psychologists, internists, family practitioners, social workers, and nurses.

The practicing psychiatrist, in our view, is vested with a difficult and sometimes peculiar responsibility—the diagnostic evaluation of psychiatric patients for the presence of occult neurologic and medical disease. No other professional from internist to nurse is in a better position by dint of training and clinical experience to make these assessments. This book is designed to provide a systematic review of these major diagnostic areas.

Ironically, despite a fairly large clinical review and book literature concerning this borderland region of clinical medicine where psychiatry, general medicine, and neurology co-mingle, there are few reference works that are organized according to the psychiatrist's experience. Thus, most of such works are organized according to various medical and neurologic syndromes, diagnoses, or physiologic systems, followed by a catalogue of behavioral phenomena which have been described in association. This is not the way psychiatry works! Mental health clinicians do not typically encounter patients who arrive tagged with their medical and neurologic diagnoses. These clinicians encounter patients who have major psychiatric syndromes, and it is for the mental health practitioners to reason from the behavior to the physiological pathologies which are reasonably likely.

We have organized our book according to the common, major psychiatric syndromes—major depression, paranoid psychosis, and others. These are the phenomena which practicing psychiatrists encounter. For each such syndrome, we attempt to provide a practical review of those medical or neurologic diseases which are likely to be co-associated, and of how the psychiatric clinician might efficiently evaluate these possibilities. We have purposefully *not* presented exhaustive lists of medical syndromes, but rather have discussed those which are likely to be encountered in practice. No disease is discussed in this book which has not been encountered within the respective practices of the authors, one of whom is a psychiatrist, one an internist, and one a neurologist. All of the clinical clues, findings, and investigations have received corroboration in our collective experience. The scientific literature of quality is sparse in these areas, but we have attempted to complement our experience with appropriate reviews.

We hope that our efforts in this book prove useful to those who care for patients from the perspective of the most difficult medical specialty: general psychiatry.

R. B. Schiffer
R. F. Klein
R. C. Sider

*Rochester, New York*

# Acknowledgments

Many people through our years of mutual experience have helped shape the ideas which we have put forth in this book. Our patients first and last have been our best teachers. They have shared with us the meanings of their experiences to the best of their abilities, and in attempting to help them we have learned from them. Our students have helped to rescue us from dogma and complacency through their questions and their ingenuous observations. We hope that in this book we have been able to give them something back that might enrich and deepen the clinical education process in psychiatry. Our teachers at the University of Rochester, especially John Romano and George Engel, have through the years helped us to become constructively curious concerning the strange distance between physical and mental life. Many of the ideas in this book have emerged from our shared mentorships with these two men. Dr. Robert Joynt has been the source or near-source of many of the aphorisms we have included in this book as clinical rules. Drs. Erwin Koranyi and William Lishman have inspired us by their example of scholarship, teaching, and clinical care. Cherie Rynerson and Cynthia O'Keefe have tirelessly and patiently provided the manuscript assistance necessary to produce the final words for the book.

# Contents

# The Medical Evaluation of Psychiatric Patients

# Introduction

> No single psychiatric symptom exists that cannot at times be caused or aggravated by various physical illnesses.
>
> *Erwin Koranyi, 1979*

The reader will be pleased to learn that in this book we have not attempted to solve the really difficult problems confronting psychiatry today. Mind–body connections, conceptual models for psychiatric practice, competing and conflicting paradigms, interdisciplinary competitions and rivalries—these and other issues all affect how psychiatrists practice. But we have discussed these thorny questions only briefly in the opening chapter with regard to their bearing on psychiatrists' involvement in the medical assessment of their patients.

What we have attempted to do is to provide a practical and useful compendium of those neurologic and medical illnesses that are most likely to become entangled clinically with the major psychiatric syndromes. We cannot say for certain that psychiatric patients today are physically sicker than in previous years, but it is certain that physical illnesses are common among our patients. It is also true that some physical illnesses are more common than others among psychiatric patients. The reasons for this must be quite interesting, but we have not considered them here. What we have done is to review those physical illnesses that have been most commonly associated with each of the major psychiatric syndromes and to outline a practical approach to their diagnostic evaluation.

The organization of Chapters 5–9 of the book is the organization provided by the major psychiatric syndromes: the psychoses, affective disorders, and anxiety disorders. After all, the psychiatrist begins clinically with the findings of the mental status examination, and his or her clinical reasoning moves on from there. In similar fashion, we have arranged each chapter around a major mental status finding and moved from there to discuss the most commonly associated physical illnesses.

Because we have designed this book as a useful guide for the practicing psychiatrist, we have had to sacrifice some depth and detail. Rare physical disorders have not been given much space, nor have those physical disorders that are no more common among psychiatric patients than among other patient populations. The inevitable result has been a clinical guide that remains incomplete. However, it has not been our goal to provide a textbook of internal medicine or neurology for psychiatrists. Our hope is that those psychiatrists who wish to include a probing search for the most likely medical syndromes among their patients will find this book a good beginning.

# 1

# Psychiatry and Physical Assessment

> Psyche and body, I suggest, react sympathetically upon each other; a change in the state of the psyche produces a change in the shape of the body, and conversely: a change in the shape of the body produces a change in the state of the psyche.
>
> *Aristotle*

Psychiatrists seldom include systematic physical assessment in their clinical practice. Patterson (1978), in a survey of psychiatrists trained at a California university center, reported that in office settings 85% seldom or never performed a physical examination as part of their initial evaluation. Of the minority who did, younger psychiatrists were much more highly represented than their older colleagues. McIntyre and Romano (1977) reported similar results in a survey of psychiatrists in Rochester, New York. They found that only 13% of full- and part-time faculty do an initial physical examination upon their inpatients and only 8% upon their outpatients.

There is a certain paradox in this fact. Psychiatrists have all survived the rigors of medical school. At considerable cost during those 4 years, they have learned impressive volumes of medical facts and mastered essential clinical skills. And at the core of the physician's identity lies the ritual of the physical exam. Among all the professions, doctors are unique in their competence, legal sanction, and societal privilege to touch and care for the human body. Moreover, in this era of role boundary diffusion among the mental health disciplines, psychiatry's role-specific status is most securely based on its frequently claimed but less frequently practiced competence in the biological aspects of diagnosis and treatment of mental disorders. Yet the evidence unequivocally documents psychiatrists' neglect of physical assessment in their clinical work.

Although it is clear how most psychiatrists actually behave with regard to physical assessment, what the profession ought to do about it is a topic of spirited debate. In the past decade, a number of authors have called attention to the frequency of previously undiagnosed physical illness among psychiatric patients (to be discussed in detail in Chapter 2), the clinical obligation of psychiatrists to assess physical factors in their evaluation of patients, and the feasibility of doing so as part of a routine "psychiatric physical exam" (Koranyi, 1979; Hall *et al.*, 1980, 1981; Summers *et al.*, 1981a,b). In contrast to their actual practice, 94% of the same psychiatrists surveyed by McIntyre and Romano stated that they believe the physical examination is sometimes or frequently useful in clinical management, particularly when the patient is receiving medication.

Others have defended the status quo, arguing that there are compelling practical and technical reasons why psychiatrists should not routinely perform physical examinations on their patients (Brown and Zinberg, 1982; Brodsky, 1970). While upholding the importance of physical assessment in the evaluation of many psychiatric patients, they believe it is best performed by another physician with whom the psychiatrist is in close contact. Current psychiatry textbooks appear thoroughly ambivalent on the issue of physical assessment, particularly the physical exam. One text devotes a single sentence to the topic (Strayhorn, 1982). Another provides a more complete, balanced discussion but begins with the advisory, "When a physical examination is indicated, for practical reasons it is usually most convenient that it be performed by an internist or family practitioner" (Kaplan and Sadock, 1985). Before examining these issues in more detail, we will consider how the present situation came about, because it is surely not by accident that psychiatrists are the only physician group for whom physical assessment of their patients is frequently overlooked.

## MEDICINE'S LEGACY

In classical times, Greek medicine was mainly somatic in orientation, a manifestation of the profession's materialist and empiricist bent. The Hippocratics created the first classification of mental disorder, including epilepsy, mania, melancholia, and paranoia. They rejected mystical theories regarding these syndromes and attributed the underlying etiology to humoral (i.e., physical) factors. In doing so, they steered Greek medicine away from the study of the mind and the use of specifically psychological therapies. Lain-Entralgo (1970) observed that although a relatively sophisticated understanding of psychotherapy is implicit in the work of the major Greek philosophers, "The Hippocratic physicians, the physicians continuing Hippocrates' work, were not wise enough to take up and make their own the legacy from Plato."

Three centuries later, the Roman philosopher Cicero asked, "Why for the care and maintenance of the body, there has been devised an art . . . whilst on the other hand the need of an art of healing for the soul has not been felt so deeply . . . nor has it been studied so closely'' (Alexander and Selesnick, 1966). Both Greek and Roman medicine acknowledged that the psyche and soma were related, that disturbance in one could produce disequilibrium in the other, and that there were clinically significant conditions that had to be appreciated as psychosomatic. But a means of effectively integrating the understanding of soul and body in theory and clinical practice was a challenge not solved by our professional progenitors of classical times.

Theodore Brown (1985) documents that by the time of Descartes there was a medical and philosophical literature describing psychosomatic and somatopsychic relationships. But extending well into the 18th century, the mentally ill were commonly regarded with fear, and the etiologies of their disorders were ascribed to a variety of natural, demonologic, and mystical forces. The vast majority of physicians were not concerned with the care of these patients. The European and American reforms of the 18th and 19th centuries were influential in humanizing these patients' treatment and subjecting their study to the methods of empirical science. But even then, the mentally ill continued to be housed in facilities entirely separate from general teaching hospitals, where, until this century, no designated psychiatric beds were available. Their care was in the hands of the alienists, a small group of atypical physicians who worked in relative isolation from their medical colleagues.

Edward Shorter (1985) proposes a classification of three successive historical periods and describes the prototypic physician for each. In the first, the traditional physician (before 1880) had neither access to modern ideas regarding psychogenic factors in the etiology of disease nor a scientific understanding of pathogenesis or therapeutics. Rather, the physician carried forward concepts linking psychic and somatic processes from classical and neoclassical times. Shorter's second period (1880–1950) is that of the modern physician. During this stage, he documents the increasing sophistication in the understanding of psychological factors in disease, the coining of the term ''psychosomatic'' in the 1930s, and the discovery of the placebo effort. Moreover, armed for the first time with high status and a scientific knowledge of disease pathogenesis, physicians were well placed to inspire the confidence of their patients, thereby increasing their powers of suggestion. Also, because physicians of this period were able to conduct their clinical consultations in a friendly, leisurely manner, the psychological benefits of their interventions were maximized.

Shorter contends that these psychologically beneficial aspects of medical care have deteriorated substantially in the past 35 years, during the third stage, that of the postmodern physician (1950 to the present). This period is characterized by the triumph of the biochemical model of disease with its exclusive focus on organic processes, a consequent depersonalized style in the physician–

patient relationship, and hurried clinical encounters because of the tight rationing of physicians' time. Shorter concludes by observing that, in the hands of contemporary postmodern physicians, the prognosis for patients with psychoneurotic and psychosomatic illnesses is significantly worse that it was 40 years ago. Stanley Reiser (1978) has persuasively linked these changes to the growing influence of technology in medicine—the extension or replacement of physicians with machines. Reiser, too, is disquieted by the reciprocal loss of attention to the medical interview, the history, the "human" factors in illness, which results from this technical, mechanical focus.

We conclude, then, that Western medicine has been characterized by a relative neglect of patients with psychological disorders but a long-standing appreciation of somatopsychic interactions. Recent decades, however, mark a period in which American physicians have become progressively more biotechnical in their orientation, thereby diminishing their earlier appreciation of mind/body links in health and illness. And it was from within this historical medical context that psychiatry emerged.

## EVOLUTION OF MODERN PSYCHIATRY

Modern psychiatry developed between 1775 and 1900, the product of two ideologically disparate parents: the organicists on the one hand and the dynamicists on the other. The views of the former are illustrated by the American Benjamin Rush, who wrote in 1812, "The cause of madness is ceded primarily in the blood vessels of the brain . . ." (Rush, 1962). In 1845, in Germany, Wilheim Griesinger stated that "although in many cases this (brain damage) cannot be ocularly demonstrated by pathological anatomy, still on physiological grounds it is universally admitted" (Alexander and Selesnick, 1966). Grounded on the empirical methods of science and buttressed by the success of medical pathology and bacteriology, the organicists anticipated the time when identifiable specific disorders of brain function and structure would solve the etiologic enigma of psychiatric illness.

At the end of the 19th century, no one exemplified the organicist approach better than Emil Kraepelin, for whom painstaking clinical description of mental symptomatology, natural history, careful physical and neurological assessment, and, ultimately, postmortem examination was the one sure method for advancing psychiatry as a scientific clinical discipline (Kraepelin, 1923, 1971). Throughout his writings, the etiology of mental disorders is attributed to organic factors: "intoxifications," "disease of the brain," "morbid constitution," "hereditary degeneracy." Only in the cases of three neurotic disorders—hysterical insanity, traumatic neurosis, and dread neurosis—does he impute purely psychogenic causes.

Within the organicist paradigm, psychopathology is conceived as a manifestation of biological disease. Therefore, the clinician's search for biological signs is always a positive search and physical assessment an integral part of the clinical workup. It was a source of continuing frustration that specific physical correlates for the major psychiatric syndromes were so frequently lacking. But for the organicists, the appropriate response was not to abandon physical assessment but rather to redouble their investigative efforts to discover the erstwhile elusive biological markers.

It is historically noteworthy that the organicists, so influential in Europe at the turn of the century, should not have prevailed in America. Although the organic paradigm always enjoyed professional support in the New World, the first half of this century saw the dynamicists overshadowing their rivals in terms of influence and popularity. The reasons are surely complex. But among them we include the pluralism, pragmatism, and optimism of the American intellectual and social climate. Here the organicists' pessimistic prognosis for mental disorders fit poorly with the abiding faith in progress deep in the American psyche. Moreover, American universities and medical schools, unfettered by the academic conservatism and hierarchical control of European centers, provided a receptive soil in which to nourish the theorists and practitioners of the new dynamic psychiatry. As we shall see, in America, when the psychodynamic paradigm achieved dominance, physical assessment moved to the periphery of the psychiatrist's clinical practice.

Psychiatry's other progenitor, the dynamic school, can be traced to Franz Anton Mesmer (Ellenberger, 1970). In 1775, he became a European sensation as the discoverer of "animal magnetism." Mesmer's claim that he could harness this cosmic source of energy for therapeutic purposes resulted in a number of dramatic cures of mental patients. A highly controversial figure, he was ultimately discredited by a French Royal Commission which found that Mesmer had provided no evidence for his claim to have discovered a "magnetic fluid" responsible for human health and illness. Historically, his importance inheres in his utilization of hypnotic methods and the route to the unconscious these methods provided. He effectively and dramatically utilized a novel explanatory theory, personal charisma, and the power of suggestion to heal a variety of mental disorders. For Mesmer, the traditional methods of physical assessment were of no use, since, to quote his famous aphorism, "There is only one illness and one healing."

During the second half of the 19th century, medical progress made possible for the first time reliable differential diagnosis between psychogenic and organic disorders. The great neurologist Jean Martin Charcot both illustrated and advanced this achievement (Ellenberger, 1970). Through careful examination and phenomenologic description, he was able to positively diagnose hysterical seizures, paralyses, and amnesias. In distinguishing organic from psychogenic illness, Charcot used the physical exam in a novel way, as a negative screen. Psychogenic illness was diagnosed when phenomenologically characteristic symptoms were observed in a patient without neurological signs of organic disease. By enabling the examiner to rule out the presence of underlying biological disease, he could then be assured that the symptoms were fundamentally psychic phenomena explainable in psychological terms. As we shall see, today's psychiatric clinicians think as Charcot thought in regard to physical assessment.

## SIGMUND FREUD

Because of his decisive impact on modern psychiatry, particularly in America, we now consider Charcot's pupil, Sigmund Freud, and the evolution of his views regarding physical assessment. Freud began his professional career as a neurologist and neuropathologist for whom sophisticated, comprehensive physical assessment was integral to his scientific and clinical work. But early in his career he had come under the influence of Breuer, had learned from him the cathartic technique, and was progressively enamored of psychic phenomena in his patients. Over the next 30 years (1895–1925), Freud's interest in the biology of mental illness progressively diminished, and he came to view himself less and less as a physician. He also experienced a growing distance between himself and the medical establishment and ultimately declared psychoanalysis not to be part of medicine.

An early turning point occurred on April 21, 1896, when Freud read a paper before his medical colleagues at the Society for Psychiatry and Neurology in Vienna, titled "The Aetiology of Hysteria" (Freud, 1962). In this paper Freud outlined his seduction theory of neurosis, that hysteria had its origins in actual traumatic sexual experience during childhood. The impact of this revolutionary theory on his colleagues is illustrated by Krafft-Ebing, who is said to have commented, "It sounds like a scientific fairy tale" (Masson, 1984). Thereafter, Freud never felt completely at home among nonpsychoanalytic physicians and sought to build the psychoanalytic movement outside the framework of academic medicine.

With the further elaboration of psychoanalytic theory and technique, the patient's body and biological processes receded further into the background as the mind and its dynamic vicissitudes came to occupy center stage. Between 1895 and 1904, Freud modified his technique so that although the patient still reclined on a couch, he was no longer required to close his eyes. The doctor, for his part, now sat on a chair behind the patient's range of vision and dispensed with pressing his hand on the patient's forehead. The method of free association now prevailed. It was no longer necessary to touch the patient's body for therapeutic purposes. It was not until 1924, however, that Freud wrote specifically about the issue of the physical assessment of psychoanalytic patients (Freud, 1959). Here he insisted on a screening medical evaluation of the prospective analysand by a physician prior to beginning analysis. Although not stated explicitly, it appears from the context to be permissible but not recommended for the analyst himself to perform the examination if he is also a physician. "I allow—no, I insist—that in every case which is under consideration for analysis the diagnosis shall be established first by a doctor." Freud was keenly aware that physical illness could masquerade as psychoneurosis and that competent medical assessment was therefore necessary in all cases to arrive at the correct diagnosis.

Once analysis had begun, he was firm that all concurrent medical concerns ought to be referred to a medical consultant. He provides three reasons for this view: "In the first place it is not a good plan for a combination of organic and psychological treatments to be carried out by one and the same person. Secondly, the relation in the transference may make it inadvisable for the analyst to examine the patient physically. And thirdly, the analyst has every reason for doubting whether he is unprejudiced, since his interests are directed so intensely to the physical factors."

Under closer examination, Freud's arguments are tantalizingly abbreviated. What does he mean, for example, by his first reason, that "it is not a good plan for a combination of organic and psychological treatments to be carried out by one and the same person?" There is the suggestion here of inherent incompatibility, that the perspective and methods the physician utilizes for one domain are unsuitable or even, perhaps, counterproductive when used for the other. Freud intimates an irreducible dualism in clinical therapeutics. Elsewhere, in commenting on the training of psychoanalysts, Freud is quite explicit: "In his medical school a doctor receives a training which is more or less opposite of what he would need as preparation for psychoanalysis . . . in itself, every science is one-sided. . . . Psychoanalysis is certainly quite particularly one-sided, as being the science of the mental unconscious. We must not therefore dispute to the medical sciences their right to be one-sided" (Freud, 1959). For Freud there could be no comprehensive physician–psychoanalyst. We may choose to treat medically or psychoanalytically, but choose we must, for we cannot do both simultaneously.

His second argument, although again very brief, is more specific. Here Freud regards physical examination as possibly disruptive to the "relation in the transference." How might this be so? Technical, therapist, and patient dynamics may be affected. From the technical side, Freud had prescribed an impassive, reflective posture for the analyst who should "follow the surgeon in regard to emotional coldness toward the patient and that his concern should be to act as a mirror reflecting for the patient what he shows to the analyst while the analyst remains opaque'' (Freud, 1958). Examining patients in the course of analysis would involve breaking out of this self-imposed role, thereby possibly contaminating the analytic field.

Freud may also have been concerned about countertransference risks, particularly of an erotic nature. During the same period, his close friend and collaborator, Sandor Ferenczi, was publishing a series of controversial papers in which he proposed certain modifications of psychoanalytic technique. These involved the recommendation that the analyst provide the patient with actual therapeutic experiences, not merely insight. This included allowing patients to sit on his lap and even to be kissed. In a charming reply to Ferenczi, Freud gently reproves him, not, he insists, because of ''prudishness or from consideration of bourgeois convention'' but rather because of the license this may appear to give to even more radical followers (Masson, 1984). Perhaps for Freud the place to draw the line was at a handshake. Physical assessment would then be off limits. From the patient's side we can speculate that Freud feared the development of somaticizing, dependent, and/or erotic transference dynamics should the analyst indulge in physical assessment during the course of psychoanalysis.

Freud's third reason, that the analyst is a prejudiced clinical observer since his interests are directed so intensely to the physical factors, appears to be a prudent caution. Psychoanalytic work requires focus and concentration. The domain of psychic life is complex and demanding enough. Why, he suggests, try in addition to be a second-rate internist? The result, he predicts, will be a reduction in skillfulness at both levels. This strikes us as an important issue. It is surely true that to conceive of patient symptoms and verbal productions in analytic terms is to do so within a wholly mentalistic framework. But it begs the more fundamental question, which remains, ''When and under what circumstances is the biological framework useful in understanding mental and behavioral symptomatology?''

## TWENTIETH-CENTURY AMERICAN PSYCHIATRY

Early in this century, American psychiatry struggled ambivalently with psychiatrists' role vis-à-vis medicine and physical assessment. On the one hand, the American Psychoanalytic Association, under the leadership of Abraham Brill, insisted, in opposition to Freud, on the requirement of the M.D. degree for all candidates for psychoanalytic training. But it is difficult to see this as anything but a political device for securing quality control and high professional status. With the advent of Naziism in the 1930s, a large number of leading European psychoanalysts emigrated to the United States, establishing themselves in psychoanalytic institutes and universities. By the 1940s and 1950s, many university departments of psychiatry were heavily staffed by psychoanalysts. Although studies in the biology of psychiatric disorders were receiving attention, and some somatic treatments, particularly ECT, had established legitimacy, the predominant theoretical orientation in American psychiatry was psychodynamic. The modern era of psychopharmacology and neurobiology had scarcely dawned. Most psychiatrists had little theoretical or therapeutic incentive to pursue the physical investigation of their patients. American psychiatrists remained physicians, but physicians of a largely noncorporeal organ—the mind.

Harry Stack Sullivan, a progressive and prominent, if unorthodox, American psychoanalyst and theorist through the 1930s and 1940s, illustrates the mood of the times (Sullivan, 1940). A major student of the psychoses, his theories linked psychiatry far more closely with the social than with the biological sciences, as indicated in his observation of the " 'mesalliance' of psychiatry and neurology." His close friend, anthropologist Edward Sapir, was outspoken in his opinion that psychiatrists had found their medical and biological training of no use in their practice but, because they longed to be accepted as medicine men, were restrained from turning to their natural home in the social sciences (Sapir, 1932).

The move away from the biological was far from unanimous, however. An early and influential advocate for a comprehensive, psychobiological psychiatry was Adolf Meyer who, in 1918, published a detailed, systematic approach to physical assessment as an integral part of the clinical workup (Meyer, 1951). Karl Menninger, psychoanalyst though he was, also contended for the importance of the physical exam and emphasized its potential therapeutic value: "It may constitute one of the most important steps in therapy . . . sometimes it is indeed the keystone of the therapeutic relationship" (Menninger, 1952). More recently, the debate over the internship requirement for psychiatric training, hotly debated during the decade 1967–77, illustrates the continuation into the present of psychiatry's ambivalence about its role in regard to the physical. Spurred by the Millis Commission report of 1966, which recommended abolishing free-standing internships prior to graduate residency training, the American Board of Psychiatry and Neurology (ABPN) in 1970 dropped the internship requirement for psychiatry residency training, thus shortening the minimal residency requirement to 3 years from 4. John Romano, at that time standing virtually alone, opposed this change, labeling it "an act of regression" and citing, among other concerns, the risk of weakening the psychiatrist's perception of self as a physician and the loss of practical clinical skills (Romano, 1970). In 1977, the ABPN reversed itself, reinstating an internship requirement, but this time mandating a minimum of only 4 months in a nonpsychiatric clinical setting. The most recent revision of the ABPN requirements, effective July 1, 1987, requires 2 months in neurology as well, raising the total nonpsychiatric time for residency training in psychiatry to 6 months.

Currently, the debate about psychiatry's future place in medicine and the use of the biological perspective in diagnosis and therapeutics shows evidence of heating up. What has been labeled psychiatry's biological revolution has, since the 1950s, had growing impact on the profession. Discoveries in the genetics, neurobiology, and natural history of mental disorder and rapid advances in psychopharmacology have all contributed to a substantial reexamination of the requisite knowledge base, skills, and methods appropriate to contemporary practice. Perhaps the most radical position has been that taken by Detre, who, in a polemical paper, argues passionately for the abandonment of the "false boundary between mind and brain" and the combining of "neurology and psychiatry into a new career path leading to specialization in clinical neuroscience" (Detre, 1987). Such trainees, no doubt, would be highly sophisticated practitioners of physical assessment.

From this brief historical survey, three observations are in order. First, the actual practice of most psychiatrists in regard to physical assessment reflects adherence to the views of the dynamic school as developed by Freud in his elaboration of the psychoanalytic method. That is, although physical assessment is important in principle, it is preferable that it be done by another physician. But beyond its dubious status as a nonessential part of psychiatrists' professional responsibility, physical assessment is seen as foreign and possibly counterproductive to their central mission.

Second, physical assessment is regarded as a negative rather than positive aid to diagnosis and treatment. The purpose of physical assessment is to rule out organic disease. When the medical evaluation is negative, the psychiatrist is assured that his prospective patient is bona fide psychiatric. Third, the biological revolution in psychiatry appears to have had far more impact on psychiatrists' therapeutic than on their diagnostic practice. Their readiness to appropriate the advances of clinical psychopharmacology has not translated into a similar degree of attention to the biological aspects of patient assessment. This discrepancy indicates that the biological revolution is, at this point, far from complete. We conclude that psychiatrists think and behave in regard to the soma in a way that is the obverse of that of the remainder of their medical colleagues. That is, in spite of sincere attempts by both groups, each has fallen to one side of the mind/body split with a consequent lack on either side of an inclusive vision.

## PSYCHIATRISTS' OBJECTIONS TO PERFORMING PHYSICAL ASSESSMENT

Five reasons are cited in the literature in defense of psychiatrists' present practice regarding physical assessment. First is the question of competence. Is it reasonable to expect clinical psychiatrists to perform physical examinations with the requisite skill? Although this is an eminently researchable question, the definitive study has yet to be done. A significant fraction of psychiatrists admit, however, not feeling competent in this regard. In Patterson's survey, 53% reported feelings of incompetence. In McIntyre and Romano's study, 32% of younger psychiatrists and 43% of older psychiatrists reported similar feelings. But skill in physical assessment can only be assessed in terms of an inferred standard. Anderson (1980), while acknowledging that psychiatrists will not auscultate the heart with the skill of a cardiologist, nonetheless asserts that in taking vital signs they are fully proficient. He also argues that the frequency with which they see subtle changes in autonomic and extrapyramidal function due to psychotropic drug side effects suggests that with practice they could become highly skilled in these areas of physical assessment as well.

Only one study, that of Summers *et al.* (1981a), reports empirically on the physical findings resulting from the use of a "psychiatric physical exam." Three examiners, one a psychiatrist and the other two psychiatrists/internists, examined an unselected sample of 75 psychiatric patients (Summers *et al.*, 1981a). An average of 5.3 "new" and 2.8 "old" physical findings per patient were found, with the psychiatrist finding somewhat fewer than his two colleagues. In a substantial fraction of cases, the physical findings were of diagnostic and therapeutic importance. Consequently, the authors conclude by recommending that the physical examination of psychiatric patients is best done by the psychiatrist, "as it may lead to confirmation of known psychiatric illness or consideration of an unsuspected psychiatric illness." We note here that competence in physical assessment is a "state" rather than "trait" characteristic. All psychiatrists were competent in physical assessment at one time, or they should not have been successful as medical students and house staff. To regain and maintain the competence requires, like any other clinical skill that has atrophied from disuse, appropriate retraining and consistent practice.

Second, some contend that physical assessment is not an efficient use of the psychiatrist's time. Such was the case with 58% of Patterson's respondents, who had another physician perform the physical exam to save time. A related aspect of efficiency is the expected yield of helpful information for time invested. But if a truly integrated, comprehensive assessment is the goal of a psychiatric evaluation, it is hardly efficient to stop halfway or to call on another physician to finish the job. Moreover, qualitatively different clinical data may be elicited from such a comprehensive approach.

Physical examination does take time. In their report, Summers *et al.* (1981a) found that the psychiatrist averaged about 20 min and the psychiatrist/internist about 15 min for a systematic but rudimentary "psychiatric physical exam." The yield of positive physical findings from these examinations, however, as reported in detail in Chapter 2, is remarkably high. A credible case can be made, therefore, that 20 min spent in physical assessment is as efficient a practice as any other component of comprehensive psychiatric evaluation.

Third is the pragmatic issue of availability of physical examination facilities. Physical assessment requires an examining table, appropriate instruments, and privacy safeguards. Few psychiatrists' offices are appropriately equipped. In a private office setting, the psychiatrist has three practical choices: install such equipment, utilize an equipped office elsewhere for physical examinations, or modify the physical exam to one that can be done with the patient in a sitting position and without disrobing. Admittedly, each of these options entails costs in terms of time, expense, or completeness. But for the large number of psychiatrists now practicing in general or psychiatric hospitals, multispecialty clinics, or community mental health centers, examination rooms may already be available or relatively easily secured. Ultimately, however, securing appropriate facilities for physical assessment is a secondary matter. Fundamental is the judgment whether physical examination is a necessary or optional component of modern psychiatric practice.

Fourth is the question of role dissonance. Brown and Zinberg (1982) have commented that when patients consult health practitioners, they come with already preformed expectations regarding reciprocal role-appropriate behaviors. Patients voluntarily consulting a psychiatrist, for example, "have already made the fundamental choice to define their problems at least partly in psychological terms." Conversely, the patient who consults a physician "usually wants to have his or her complaint taken at face value." Similar expectations may also apply in terms of the psychiatrist's role identity. Those who were trained and now practice almost exclusively within a mentalistic model may experience themselves "in role" only when talking to patients and quite out of role when physically examining them. These reciprocally reinforcing role expectations constitute a source of inertial energy maintaining the status quo. But unpublished data of our own, which we will summarize below, suggest that both psychiatrists and patients may be quite malleable in this regard.

The fifth objection is potentially the most important: that physical assessment may actually be harmful. Recall our discussion of Freud's concerns cited earlier in this chapter. If harm is to be done, two possible mechanisms seem most likely. First, might physical assessment increase the risk of sexual intimacy? Erikson (1950) has observed that integrated sharing on both a physical and mental level is generally confined to a mutual love relationship. On this basis, Brown and Zinberg (1982) argue that psychiatrists' "awareness of problems or emotional discomfort that could result from extreme intimacy—exceeding that already inherent in either intense psychological or medical work alone—may deter the integration of psychological and physical care." Kardener (1974), in a discussion of sexual intimacy in the physician–patient relationship, similarly believes that psychiatrists' practice of not performing a physical exam "may serve as (a) factor that militates against erotic involvement."

Although this argument is plausible, it is asserted in the absence of supporting data. The risk of sexual behavior, although difficult to reliably measure, does not appear to be significantly different across medical specialties. Moreover, the evidence suggests that for the large majority of physicians of any specialty, appropriate ethical standards are maintained. In psychiatric practice, it may also be true that the distinctly unromantic procedure of the physical examination will inhibit the potential eroticization of the relationship, in contrast to a strictly psychotherapeutic approach, in which physical fantasies may abound. Still, we agree with Menninger (1952) that in certain cases, best left to the discretion of the individual psychiatrist, the performance of a physical examination may be relatively contraindicated because of the possibility of heightening erotic temptations.

A more general objection is that physical assessment may interfere with the patient's development of a therapeutic relationship. This view is credible within the constraints of classical psychoanalysis. But for the vast majority of psychiatric patients, it is equally plausible to believe that physical assessment may enhance the therapeutic relationship. In an unpublished study, the authors of this book assigned unselected new psychiatric outpatients at a university community mental health center to participating PGY-III psychiatric residents for initial evaluation. Randomly, half the patient group was assigned to a "no physical examination" protocol, the other half to a protocol including the physical examination. Patients were separately interviewed by a faculty investigator within 3 weeks of their initial evaluation and again after 6 months. During these interviews, the patient's global satisfaction was measured with the Medical Interview Satisfaction Scale. Although the numbers were small ($n = 10$), the findings are suggestive. First, all of the patients who were physically examined responded that the physical examination either had no effect or had enhanced their confidence in and satisfaction with the treating physician. Virtually all of the patients, whether or not they were in the physical examination group, endorsed physical examination as an appropriate and potentially beneficial part of psychiatric evaluation.

The participating residents similarly found that performing a physical examination in no case impeded the development of a psychotherapeutic relationship. In some cases, they believed the physical examination had increased their psychological understanding of the patient and had substantially benefited the therapeutic relationship. Two brief vignettes are instructive.

## Case 1: The Neurotic with a Penile Injury

A 28-year-old man was self-referred to the residents' clinic at Strong Memorial Hospital after a psychotherapeutic failure experience at a community hospital. His complaints included a somewhat vague and long-standing history of anxious and depressive feelings, causing him some difficulty in relationships with women. His work achievements had proceeded reasonably well, however, and he was employed as an administrator at a local radio station at the time of referral. He was randomized to physical examination by his similar-aged male PG-III psychiatry resident.

During the rectal–genital portion of the examination, penile scarring and deformity was noted. The patient related at this time that he had accidentally injured his penis during adolescence while masturbating with a glass object. He further acknowledged that he had not felt able to discuss this with his previous psychotherapist, even though the knowledge of the penile scarring underlay many of his brooding and anxious emotions.

At the time of the examination, both the resident therapist and the faculty observer had felt quite uncomfortable—as if they had invaded the privacy of this young man. In recording the data obtained during the immediate postexamination conference, both expressed a fear that this exam had harmed the patient. The faculty observer recorded his reassurance that informed consents were obtained prior to the conduct of the examinations.

At the 6-month review of psychotherapeutic progress, however, quite a different reaction had become apparent on the part of the patient. He had expressed considerable relief during weekly sessions after the examination, as well as a productive self-examination of his feelings of guilt and inferiority over the penile injury. Considerable symptomatic improvement had occurred during the subsequent 6 months. The judgment of the faculty observer and the resident therapist was that the physical examination had caused the psychiatrists to feel considerably more uncomfortable than the patient, for whose psychotherapy it had proved facilitating.

## Case 2: The Chronic Schizophrenic Who Lifts Weights

A 35-year-old man with a diagnosis of chronic undifferentiated schizophrenia was "rotated" to one of the psychiatric residents in our study after his previous resident graduated. Chronic antipsychotic medication was prescribed for this patient, with variable compliance. He lived in a supervised residence home and came for brief medication checks every 2 months. He was randomized to receive a physical examination.

During the examination of the motor system, it became clear that the patient was quite well muscled, which observation the resident made explicitly. The patient added that he lifted weights regularly at his group home. No other positive findings were made on this patient, and neither resident nor faculty observer thought that anything of importance had transpired during the examination.

Again, during the 6-month review, it became apparent that something *had* happened from the patient's perspective. Although his history was one of being somewhat distant and unengaged from his therapist, the patient had actively related to the psychiatric resident around this issue of body building. He made it clear that his self-esteem had risen substantially as a result of the examiner's observations concerning his musculature and that his physique was one of his few "assets." Both faculty observer and resident concluded that a supportive psychotherapeutic bond had begun, quite unintentionally, during the examination.

Our data suggest, admittedly on the basis of a small sample, that the warnings regarding potential harm resulting from the psychiatric physical exam may have been exaggerated.

## PERSONALITY AND ATTITUDINAL CHARACTERISTICS OF PSYCHIATRISTS

Yet another variable may be important in understanding psychiatrists' avoidance of physical assessment. It is alluded to in Patterson's survey, where 42% of his respondents reported that they "did not like performing physical exams" (Patterson, 1978). We will resist comment on the merits of determining one's clinical approach to patient evaluation on the basis of personal likes and dislikes. Instead, we discuss here the evidence that there are significant attitudinal and personality differences between psychiatrists and other physician groups that may affect their predisposition not to routinely perform physical examinations.

A number of studies concur that medical students choosing psychiatry are different from their peers and that these differences are greater than those distinguishing other specialty groups (Eagle and Marcos, 1980). Because these dissimilarities antedate psychiatric training, they reflect underlying personality characteristics rather than education effects. Moreover, the nature of these differences suggests that they may help to explain why future psychiatrists are attracted to our field. Could it also shed light on their relative neglect of physical assessment? Consider the following.

Future psychiatrists are distinguished by their professional interests. They are more person-oriented, are more humanistic, score higher on "nurturance," and lean toward the interpersonal aspects of patient care (Yugit *et al.*, 1969; Sharaf *et al.*, 1968). These findings suggest that those choosing psychiatry are seeking a clinical specialty in which the psychological and relational aspects of care predominate. To oversimplify, psychiatrists are more interested and therefore derive greater satisfaction when they view their patients more as persons than as organisms. Hence, the intrinsic appeal of the biological perspective and of physical assessment is diminished.

A second set of characteristics differentiates future psychiatrists in how they think. They are more theoretically than pragmatically oriented and are more reflective, open-minded, and tolerant of ambiguity (Walton, 1969; Paiva and Haley, 1971; Matteson and Smith, 1977). Ideas and the subjective realm of human experience appear most actively to engage the minds of psychiatrists. They are more at home with process and possibility than with content and certainty. The approach of the medical physician to workup, ever searching for the definitive diagnosis, is the opposite of the average psychiatrist's more laissez-faire approach. Psychiatrists do not possess the same need to know the diagnosis. It is enough that they understand their patient's experience.

Both of the previously identified groups of characteristics plausibly explain psychiatrists' tendency to prefer the mental and personal realm over the biological. But there is a third pair of variables that suggest that a biophobic factor may also be at work, that psychiatrists may actively avoid the body and physical assessment. In a fascinating study, Livingston and Zimet (1965) found that future psychiatrists were distinguished from their peers by lower scores on "authoritarianism" but higher scores on "death anxiety." The authoritarian personality sees relationships in more power-related and hierarchical terms, is action-oriented, and comfortably assumes an executive posture. Brown and Zinberg (1982) observe that predisposition toward action and executive responsibility "fits" more naturally with the medical physician's role with physically sick patients. If psychiatrists are relatively less comfortable assuming such a role posture, they may avoid physical assessment, preferring to talk to their patients instead. Their higher scores on "death anxiety" are similarly instructive. If psychiatrists are relatively more afraid of death (this may simply reflect increased awareness of their fears), they may avoid dealing directly with that which is mortal—the body.

We do not wish to overstate the differences between psychiatrists and other physicians. There is a wide scatter in the distribution of personality variables within psychiatry, as there is throughout medicine. But we believe that psychiatrists' tendency to avoid physical assessment is not entirely due to historical, professional, educational, or social artifact. It is also a function of who psychiatrists are and why they chose their specialty. It is also possible that such selection processes may be modified over time and that the character of a specialty can change.

## THE PROBLEM OF JANUS

We turn now to the vexing issue of the nature of the human organism, the object of clinical inquiry. In our view, this constitutes the source of the most fundamental hindrance to clinicians' more balanced utilization of physical *and* psychological assessment. In doing so, we forewarn the reader that, unlike most contemporary psychiatric authors, we do not propose to abolish the mind/body enigma, either through appeal to general systems theory, a biological reductionism, or a wholly mentalistic metapsychology. We believe, as do McHugh and Slavney (1983), that the council of clinical wisdom is for psychiatrists to think and behave as practical dualists, regarding their patients both as subjects *and* objects, agents *and* organisms. This approach is required because of the bimodal character of human nature and thus of our clinical knowledge of patients. There is at present no satisfactory resolution to the mind/body problem in terms of any available monistic theory.

So far in this chapter we have repeatedly encountered the tendency of other physicians and psychiatrists to fall to one side or the other of the mind/body boundary. They do so not because of some intellectual or moral venality, but because the boundary is real and unavoidable. Human nature is two-sided. Unlike other objects of our understanding, knowledge of human beings is gained through two different avenues and yields two kinds of truth: the objective and the subjective. To apprehend patients objectively is to view them as objects among others in the phenomenal world, noting their distinguishing properties in order to allow identification, description, and classification. Eliciting physical findings is an exercise in the objective mode. Mental phenomena can also be viewed within the objective perspective. Although not palpably present, patients' thoughts and feelings are accessible to us through their verbal reports. Objectively, these are apprehended by us in terms of the forms and patterns of their occurrence. For example, when in recording the Mental State Examination we report the presence of auditory hallucinations, we are objectifying these mental experiences. Viewed in this way, symptoms and signs are objects in the natural world, and knowledge gained about them is objective knowledge. Moreover, we understand this knowledge in terms of an explanatory framework that is naturalistic (scientific). To these objects, the law of causality applies.

But we may also come to know our patients subjectively, as persons. This knowledge requires a different methodology and yields an altogether different mode of understanding. Here we attempt to know our patients as subjects, from the inside, to see them in their subjective singularity. It is only possible to do so, however, through personal engagement. We must feel our way into their experience, empathizing and thereby recreating within ourselves their subjective reality. Once "inside" in this way, we apprehend our patients' experience in terms of motives and meanings, the viscissitudes of a living, self-determining human agent. Understanding of this type takes the form of narrative, a life story.

Karl Jaspers (1964) has elucidated this distinction in terms of Erklaren (perception of causal connection) and Verstehen (perception of meaning). Habermas (1971) has contrasted these modes of knowing in terms of the difference between the natural sciences, where "an explanation requires the application of theoretical propositions to facts that are established independently through systematic observation," and the cultural sciences, where "in understanding I transpose my own self into something external in such a way that a past or foreign experience becomes present in my own." Whether one mode of knowledge is ultimately more "true" than the other and whether one mode is reducible to the other are questions well beyond the purview of this book. Here we wish to underline the inescapable two-sidedness of our knowledge of our patients and the consequence this poses for comprehensive clinical understanding.

Nemiah (1981) has illustrated the clinical impact of this issue in a candid personal account. He recalls his own failure to include the drug treatment for panic disorder in a chapter he wrote for a major textbook some years after such treatment had been demonstrated to be effective. His explanation for what he calls this "disgraceful" oversight is instructive: "There appears to be an inherent tension between biological and psychological modes of thinking. One tends to think *either* biologically *or* psychologically and it seems to be difficult to combine the two modes effectively."

We have already identified one source of Nemiah's difficulty, namely, that these are two different kinds of knowledge, but a further problem also obtains. Each domain of knowledge entails demands on the knower that are incompatible with the other. Consider first the objective mode. To understand our patients as objects, we must objectify them, that is, view them from the outside. To do so requires a detached, dispassionate posture in which our patient is depersonified. In viewing patients objectively, empathic identification and emotional arousal are counterproductive. To pursue objective knowledge effectively, we must actively suppress our human sympathies.

But it is precisely these sympathies that enable us to see with our subjective eye, for we can only know our patients from the inside by personifying them through empathic identification. Havens (1974) states his belief that it is this latter capacity which is uniquely fundamental to the psychiatrist's role: "Psychiatric practice, perhaps more than any other specialty, rests on the empathic resources of the doctor. . . . Psychiatric treatment consists, to a significant extent, of heightened receptivity."

It seems clear to us that clinicians cannot be expected simultaneously to view their patients subjectively and objectively. It is like attempting to see clearly while using both a hyperopic and myopic eye. The objective eye sees at a great distance, cool and detached, scanning the contours of the world for patterns. The subjective eye sees only at extremely close range, requiring intimate apposition to make its perceptual images visible. It is no surprise that psychiatrists and other physicians, like the child with strabismus, learn to suppress one image and to see almost exclusively with the favored eye.

Yet another aspect of the Janus problem bedevils us here. It is that there are few reliable clues to help us select which perspective to utilize in a given clinical context. The housewife who complains of debilitating headaches in the context of an unsatisfactory marriage to an infuriating husband may be suffering from unexpressed rage. But she may also have a glioma. Some symptoms—e.g., offensive olfactory hallucinations—are often associated with neuropathology. Others, such as the grief reaction experienced following the death of a loved one, we understand empathically as a human response to loss. But the remainder of this book documents that there are few reliable discriminators for a large number of psychiatric disorders. Postviral depression, thyrotoxic anxiety, and amphetamine psychosis are not phenomenologically distinct from other depressions, anxiety states, and paranoid disorders.

The converse of the absence of reliable discriminators is that any mental experience is equally well explained within both objective and subjective modes. This fundamental ambiguity is the origin of much of the endless feuding between psychiatric partisans of mentalist versus physicalist perspectives. Searching for signposts in these murky waters, psychiatrists frequently make false assumptions. These result in an increased sense of direction but are attended with greater risk of diagnostic error. Sternberg (1986) identifies four of these: that the absence of cognitive impairment rules out physical disease; that symptoms imply diagnosis; that specific physical diseases cause only one or two psychiatric syndromes; and that the presence of psychosocial stressors is sufficient to explain the patient's symptoms. Each of these assumptions is, as Sternberg notes, a false guide. Taken together, they provide a rationale for neglecting physical assessment. But it is a rationale without justification.

## A NOT-SO-MODEST PROPOSAL

In this book, we do not attempt to prescribe for the psychiatric profession as a whole or to dictate the practice patterns of individual clinicians. Indeed, our search for the operative factors hindering psychiatrists from undertaking careful physical assessment of their patients has resulted in a rather impressive list. The impediments are several, their combined effects substantial. Perhaps we would be well advised to reluctantly bless the status quo as the most realistic compromise.

Yet we cannot do so. For we believe there is a growing cadre of psychiatrists who would like to attempt the truly difficult task of comprehensive psychophysical assessment and that substantial benefits will accrue to patients and psychiatrists when this approach is utilized. First, to our patients. What could be more reassuring than to have one's psychiatrist base his or her treatment recommendations on the results of thorough psychophysical evaluation? In cases where robust physical health is documented, patient and physician are free to focus their work appropriately at the psychological level. In other cases, where physical illness is discovered, necessary steps can be taken to assure proper management for the patient's entire clinical needs, psychological and physical. Second, to the psychiatrist. Balanced psychophysical assessment can only enhance a psychiatrist's identity as a physician. It will yield increased self-confidence and accuracy in diagnosis and management while decreasing anxiety over missing potentially important diagnostic clues. Further, it will engender greater respect for psychiatrists, both from other physicians who, in their professional dialogue with them, will experience a greater degree of common ground, and from other, nonphysician mental health professionals, who will readily acknowledge the special contribution these psychiatrists can make to clinical assessment, not just to somatic therapies. Finally, in an era of increasingly vigorous cost containment, psychiatrists who practice on the basis of comprehensive psychophysical assessment will most easily document the unique value of their professional services.

For those psychiatrists choosing this course, we recommend that physical assessment, including a medical history and physical examination by the psychiatrist, be a part of the initial evaluation of each psychiatric patient, no more important but no less than the psychiatric history or the mental state exam. Every patient would then undergo both objective and subjective evaluation. If, as we believe, both perspectives cannot be simultaneously entertained, the examiner must report to obtaining first one view, then the other. Each perceptual eye must be opened alternately. This might best be done at a first and second visit. The resulting images are not unlike the figure/ground reversals of gestalt psychiatry. Although with each eye one sees the image, each is perceived quite differently.

To understand our patients as persons as well as to identify and explain the syndromic patterns of their symptoms and physical signs together comprise the mandate of this new breed of psychiatrist. But commitment to comprehensive psychophysical assessment cannot be undertaken lightly. Such a professional posture will be extraordinarily taxing, intellectually and clinically, a calling worthy of the best and the brightest. And there are corresponding dangers. If in the attempt to give physical assessment its proper place, psychiatrists neglect the psychological, then the substantial advances due to psychiatry's humanistic perspective would be tragically lost. The trick will be to keep these perspectives in dialectic balance. Slavney and McHugh (1987) observe: "Explanation is no more fundamental than understanding, nor is understanding more profound than explanation; they're only different methods with different strengths and weaknesses. As long as we continue to view human beings as object/organisms *and* subject/agents, both methods are essential to our practice." This book is aimed at the further equilibration of that balance.

## REFERENCES

Alexander, F. G., and Selesnick, S. T. *The History of Psychiatry*. New York: Harper and Row, 1966.

Anderson, W. H. The physical examination in office practice. *Am J. Psychiatry*, 1980, **137**, 1188–1192.

Brodsky, C. M. The systemic incompatibility of medical practice and psychotherapy. *Dis. Nerv. Syst.*, 1970, **31**, 597–604.

Brown, H. N., and Zinberg, N. E. Difficulties in the integration of psychological and medical practices. *Am J. Psychiatry*, 1982, **139**, 12:1576–1680.

Brown, T. M. Descartes, dualism, and psychosomatic medicine. In Bynum, W. F., Porter, R., and Shepherd, M. (Eds.): *The Anatomy of Madness: Essays in the History of Psychiatry*, Vol. 1. London: Tavistock Publications, 1985.

Detre, T. The future of psychiatry. *Am. J. Psychiatry*, 1987, **144**, 621–625.

Eagle, P. F., and Marcos, L. R. Factors in medical students' choice of psychiatry. *Am J. Psychiatry*, 1980, **137**, 423–427.

Ellenberger, H. F. *The Discovery of the Unconscious*. New York: Basic Books, 1970.

Erikson, E. H. *Childhood and Society*. New York: Norton, 1950.

Freud, S. *The Standard Edition of the Complete Psychological Works of Sigmund Freud*, Vol. XII, trans. J. Strachey. London: Hogarth, 1958.

Freud, S. *The Standard Edition of the Complete Psychological Works of Sigmund Freud*, Vol. XX, trans. J. Strachey. London: Hogarth, 1959.

Freud, S. *The Standard Edition of the Complete Psychological Works of Sigmund Freud*, Vol. III, trans. J. Strachey. London: Hogarth, 1962.

Habermas, J. *Knowledge and Human Interests*, trans. J. J. Shapiro. Boston: Beacon Press, 1971.

Hall, R. C. S., Gardner, E. R., Popkin, M. K., LeCann, A. F., and Popkin, M. K. Physical illness manifesting as psychiatric disease. II. Analysis of a state hospital inpatient population. *Arch. Gen. Psychiatry*, 1980, **37**, 989–995.

Havens, L. L. The existential use of the self. *Am. J. Psychiatry*, 1974, **131**, 1–10.

Jaspers, K. *General Psychopathology*, trans. J. Hoenig, M. N. Hamilton. Manchester, U.K.: Manchester University Press, 1964.

Kaplan, H. I., and Sadock, B. J. *Comprehensive Textbook of Psychiatry/IV*, 4th ed. Baltimore: Williams and Wilkins, 1985.

Kardener, S. H. Sex and the physician–patient relationship. *Am. J. Psychiatry*, 1974, **131**, 1134–1136.

Koranyi, E. K. Morbidity and rate of undiagnosed physical illnesses in a psychiatric clinic population. *Arch. Gen. Psychiatry*, 1979, **36**, 414–419.

Kraepelin, E. *Clinical Psychiatry*, abstracted and adapted by A. R. Diefendorf. London: Macmillan, 1923.

Kraepelin, E. *Lectures in Clinical Psychiatry*, ed. G. M. Robertson, trans. M. M. Barclay. Huntington, NY: Robert Krueger, 1971.

Lain-Entralgo, P. *The Therapy of the Word in Classical Antiquity*, trans. L. J. Rather, J. M. Sharp. New Haven, CT: Yale University Press, 1970.

Livingston, P. B., and Zimet, C. N. Death anxiety, authoritarianism, and choice of specialty in medical students. *J. Nerv. Ment. Dis.*, 1965, **140**, 222–230.

Masson, J. M. *The Assault on Truth: Freud's Suppression of the Seduction Theory*. New York: Farrar, Straus and Giroux, 1984.

Matteson, M. T., and Smith, S. V. Selection of medical specialties: Preferences versus choices. *J. Med. Educ.*, 1977, **52**, 548–554.

McHugh, P. R., and Slavney, P. R. *The Perspectives of Psychiatry*. Baltimore: Johns Hopkins University Press, 1983.

McIntyre, J. S., and Romano, J. Is there a stethoscope in the house (and is it used)? *Arch. Gen. Psychiatry*, 1977, **34**, 1147–1151.

Menninger, K. *A Manual for Psychiatric Case Study*. New York: Grune and Stratton, 1952.

Meyer, A. *The Collected Papers of Adolf Meyer*, Vol. III, ed. E. E. Winters. Baltimore, Johns Hopkins University Press, 1951.

Nemiah, J. C. The idea of a psychiatric education. *J. Psychiatr. Educ.*, 1981, **5**, 183–194.

Paiva, R. E. A., and Haley, H. B. Intellectual, personality, and environmental factors in career specialty preferences. *J. Med. Educ.*, 1971, **46**, 281–289.

Patterson, C. W. Psychiatrists and physical examinations: A survey. *Am. J. Psychiatry*, 1978, **135**, 967–968.

Reiser, S. J. *Medicine and the Reign of Technology*. Cambridge, U.K.: Cambridge University Press, 1978.

Romano, J. The elimination of the internship: An act of regression. *Am. J. Psychiatry*, 1970, **126**, 1565–1576.

Rush, B. *Medical Inquiries and Observation upon the Diseases of the Mind*. New York: Hafner, 1962.

Sapir, E. Cultural anthropology and psychiatry. *J. Abnorm. Soc. Psychol.*, 1932, **27**, 229–242.

Sharaf, J. R., Schneider, P., and Kantor, D. Psychiatric interest and its correlates among medical students. *Psychiatry*, 1968, **31**, 150–160.

Shorter, E. *Bedside Manners, the Troubled History of Doctors and Patients*. New York: Simon and Schuster, 1985.

Slavney, P. R., and McHugh, P. A. *Psychiatric Polarities, Methodology, and Practice*. Baltimore: Johns Hopkins University Press, 1987.

Sternberg, D. E. Testing for physical illness in psychiatric patients. *J. Clin. Psychiatry*, 1986, **47**, 3–9.

Strayhorn, J. M. *Foundations of Clinical Psychiatry*. Chicago: Year Book, 1982.

Sullivan, H. S. Conceptions of modern psychiatry: The first William Alanson White Memorial Lectures. *Psychiatry*, 1940, **3**, 1–117.

Summers, W. K., Munoz, R. A., and Read, M. R. The psychiatric physical examination. I. Methodology. *J. Clin. Psychiatry*, 1981a, **42**, 95–98.

Summers, W. K., Munoz, R. A., Read, M. R., and Marsh, G. M. The psychiatric physical examination. II. Findings in 75 unselected psychiatric patients. *J. Clin. Psychiatry*, 1981b, **42**, 99–102.

Walton, H. J. Personality correlates of a career interest in psychiatry. *Br. J. Psychiatry*, 1969, **115**, 211–219.

Yufit, R. I., Pollock, G. H., and Wasserman, E. Medical specialty choice and personality. I. Initial results and predictions. *Arch. Gen. Psychiatry*, 1969, **20**, 89–99.

# 2

# Physical Illness among Psychiatric Patients

> Psychiatry is the only medical specialty that demands for its backgrounding the whole of medicine because it is the only medical specialty that deals with the whole individual.
>
> *W. A. White*
> Presidential Address before the
> American Psychiatric Association, 1925

Psychiatric patients do not live as long as other people. This fact of psychiatric life was first reported early in the 20th century, and recent epidemiologic studies indicate that it continues to be true. It is a matter of central concern for all psychiatrists.

The reasons why psychiatric patients should experience reduced life expectancy are not entirely clarified. There are several possibilities. Psychiatric diseases themselves may shorten life-span for individuals and groups by mechanisms such as suicide. In addition, there may be some sort of shared vulnerability for psychiatric and general medical illnesses, so that people who have one are more likely to have the other. Such a shared vulnerability would not have to take the form of a genetic or biologic mechanism, but could as well be behaviorally mediated. There is some evidence for such a shared vulnerability, but this evidence is not as convincing as it is generally thought to be. And lastly, there may be specific links between certain general medical or neurologic diseases and various psychiatric syndromes, so that a certain number of patients with psychiatric syndromes are actually experiencing those syndromes as manifestations of an underlying medical illness.

We believe that this last area represents the realm of specific diagnostic and therapeutic expertise for psychiatrists. This book addresses itself primarily to these specific medical–psychiatric links. Since the clinical research evidence concerning these specific links is weak in many respects, however, we would like to review the data concerning the more general and nonspecific sort of association between psychiatric and medical illness. Are psychiatric patients generally "sicker" than other sorts of people?

## MEDICAL MORBIDITY AMONG PSYCHIATRIC PATIENTS

Very few have contended that it is healthy to be mentally ill. Many clinical and epidemiological reports, however, have implied a positive association between mental illness and a variety of general medical illnesses.

When psychiatric outpatients are examined carefully, it is consistently found that active medical problems are present (Hall *et al.*, 1978; Koranyi, 1979; Wynne-Davies, 1965; Browning *et al.*, 1974; Barnes *et al.*, 1983; McCarrick *et al.*, 1986). The larger series report prevalence rates of general medical problems consistently in the 40–50% range regardless of whether chronic outpatients, acute clinic patients, or emergency room patients are surveyed. Many of the medical diagnoses are neither acute nor life-threatening, such as mild hypertension or glucose intolerance, and in most of these reports the great majority of medical problems were considered incidental to the psychiatric symptomatology. Still, it is clear that at least a substantial minority of physical illnesses among psychiatric outpatients have not been previously identified by referral sources when the patients arrive at the psychiatric clinic. It is conceivable that if unidentified and untreated, these chronic medical problems could contribute over time to a reduced life expectancy among psychiatric patients.

Studies of psychiatric inpatients report similar prevalence rates for nonpsychiatric illness (Koranyi, 1982; Hall *et al.*, 1980; Wynne-Davies, 1964; Bunce *et al.*, 1982; Hoffman, 1982). Among more psychologically disturbed inpatients, there may be a greater number of psychiatric syndromes that are considered to be linked etiologically with an underlying medical illness than is the case among outpatients. Hall *et al.* (1980), for example, reported that when their group carefully assessed 100 consecutive inpatient admissions to a research psychiatric ward, they found that 46% of the patients had some previously unrecognized physical illness that was either causing or exacerbating their psychiatric symptomatology. Hoffman (1982) evaluated 215 consecutive admissions to a private medical psychiatric unit and found that 34% of the "functional" psychiatric diagnoses were changed to "organic" mental syndromes. Although there may have been some selection bias involved in these reports, we are left with summary statistics from more than 13 studies that indicate a 50% prevalence of active medical disorders among psychiatric inpatients (Bunce *et al.*, 1982).

Beyond these prevalence and incidence reports, there is some evidence that psychiatric patients tend to have more *severe* medical illnesses than would be expected simply from the demographic characteristics of the patients. Eastwood (1975), for example, conducted a case control study of patients in a general medical clinic who scored highly on the Cornell Medical Index Health Questionnaire. Compared with matched patients in the same clinic who scored low on this index of general emotional disturbance, the high-scoring group demonstrated a greater number of active medical problems and diagnoses. Using a large computer data base of Veterans Administration inpatients, Dvoredsky and Cooley (1986) reported that patients with both mental and physical diagnoses tended to have longer admissions than patients with just mental or just physical diagnoses.

There is no simple or brief explanation for this statistical association between physical and mental illness. The "Trojan horse" phenomenon undoubtedly explains some of the variance in this association. That is, there are undoubtedly a number of patients with general medical illness who enter psychiatric units because of behavioral manifestations of their illnesses. As long ago as 1936, Comroe reported a follow-up study of 100 psychiatric inpatients who had been diagnosed as "neurotic." During a 2-year follow-up period, 24 of these patients developed physical illnesses, most of which could quite plausibly be connected with the psychiatric symptomatology. We are far from certain that we are doing significantly better today with regard to diagnostic accuracy.

Other cogent objections can be made to many of these epidemiologic studies. In some reports, "organic mental syndrome" diagnoses have been included among the psychiatric disorders, which invites a tautology in connecting psychiatric and physical illness. We have mentioned selection bias as a possible factor in some studies. In other studies, relatively trivial medical diagnoses have been included, such as obesity or ST segment elevations on EKG.

Still, it is our conclusion that there is too much smoke in these reports for there not to be at least a small fire. One need not subscribe to "psychosomatic" hypotheses to accept the plausible conclusion that psychiatric patients take poor care of themselves and are generally cared for poorly by our medical system. The clinician who deals with psychiatric patients may reliably expect that from 20% to 50% of them will have active physical illnesses of varying severity (Lipowski, 1975). Vascular disease, diabetes mellitus, and endocrine disease are likely to be particularly common, but most other general medical and surgical conditions seem quite capable of appearing as well. The older the patient population with which one deals, the more likely it is that one or several concurrent physical illnesses will be encountered. And it seems reasonable to conclude that our present medical-care systems fail to ensure that physical diseases will be diagnosed and treated prior to the patient's arrival within a psychiatric setting. That is to say, psychiatric reliance upon the notion of "medical clearance" of psychiatric patients by other physicians is no longer an acceptable procedure. On the contrary, even when patients have a primary care physician, there is at least a 50% chance that one or more of their active physical problems will be undiagnosed when they arrive within psychiatry.

---

*Clinical Rule No. 2.1*: There are no psychiatric patients—only medical patients with varying degrees of psychopathology.

---

## MORTALITY STUDIES AMONG PSYCHIATRIC PATIENTS

Two questions are of special interest in the mortality studies that have been made of psychiatric patients. Is the excess mortality among such patients attributable wholly to their excess death rates from unnatural, psychiatric causes, such as suicide and accidents, or do psychiatric patients also die prematurely of more general medical illnesses? And if psychiatric patients do experience excess mortality from medical illness, are there specific diagnostic associations between medical and psychiatric diseases?

In one of the earlier studies that attempted to take into consideration the distinction between "natural" and "unnatural" causes of death, Koranyi (1977) retrospectively determined causes of death in a cohort of 2070 consecutive psychiatric outpatients. After a 3-year follow-up, he was able to ascertain 28 deaths, which occurred in the following general categories: natural causes, 13; suicide, 11; accidents, 4. Of the 13 persons who died of natural causes, eight died of vascular disease (myocardial infarction or related), and four of malignancies of various types. It is interesting to note, however, that eight of the patients who succumbed to general medical illness had received various "organic reaction" psychiatric diagnoses upon initial assessment in the psychiatric clinic. Perhaps wisely, Koranyi did not attempt a statistical comparison of the observed mortality with actuarial data for Canadian citizens. One can see that the inclusion of "organic" diagnoses within psychiatric cohorts might unfairly bias comparisons with population norms *against* death rates in the psychiatric group, since these patients, by definition, have significant medical illness.

It has been difficult to perform epidemiologic studies that are free of this built-in selection bias. One interesting approach to this problem has been the twin-study analyses obtained from data in the National Academy of Sciences–National Research Council Twin Registry (Kendler, 1986). Kendler, in this study, calculated standardized mortality ratios for patients diagnosed either "schizophrenic" or "neurotic" who had either monozygotic or dizygotic co-twins. Rates of expected mortality for persons in the registry, all of whom are U.S. veterans, were calculated from actuarial data for service veterans. Leaving aside deaths from trauma and suicide, which were predictably elevated, this study found significantly elevated mortality from all medical diseases (infection, vascular disease, malignancy) among the psychiatric patients. A further interesting finding of this study was that disease-related mortality was equal in two pairs (whether monozygotic or dizygotic) discordant for schizophrenia, and in twin pairs discordant for neurosis there was at least a trend toward elevated medical mortality among affected sibs. These data could be construed as providing evidence for a somapsyche illness link at least among the nonschizophrenic patients.

Other epidemiologic studies following large numbers of psychiatric patients have not found excessive mortality attributable to medical diseases (Eastwood *et al.*, 1982; Martin *et al.*, 1985a,b). In the prospective study of psychiatric inpatients from the University of Iowa, most of the excessive mortality could be attributed to unnatural causes (Tsuang *et al.*, 1980). These authors did report, however, that death rates from infectious diseases were excessive in the schizophrenia subgroup of patients and that excess cardiovascular deaths occurred among female manic patients. To us, these data imply at least the possibility of substandard medical care as a factor in life expectancy among some psychiatric patients.

## GENERAL POPULATION STUDIES OF PSYCHIATRIC DISEASE AND MORTALITY

Epidemiologic studies of general populations or population samples are somewhat divided concerning an association between mental illness and premature death from disease. The Lundby Study in Sweden and the 20-year follow-up of the Midtown Manhattan sample did not detect increased mortality from illness among individuals previously treated for mental illness (Rorsman *et al.*, 1982; Singer *et al.*, 1976). In a more recent analysis of the data from Stirling County, Canada, however, it was found that increased mortality from vascular disease was associated with previous affective disorder diagnoses (Murphy *et al.*, 1987).

### Psychiatric Disease-Specific Mortality

The issue of psychiatric disease-specific mortality has proved equally elusive. In a case-control study from the University of Iowa, 5412 psychiatric inpatients were followed for 2 years postdischarge (Winokur and Block, 1987). Seventy-three had died from unnatural causes during this time, and 115 from natural causes. Controls for the patients who had died were selected from next consecutive psychiatric admissions. There were no significant differences between the two groups with regard to psychiatric or medical diagnoses.

When Hoenig and Hamilton (1966) reassessed a mixed cohort of 273 psychiatric outpatients and inpatients after a 4-year period, they found that 54 deaths had occurred. When the deaths were tabulated on the basis of initial psychiatric diagnosis, three syndromes accounted for the great majority: "organic reactions," 26 deaths; affective psychoses, 11 deaths; schizophrenia, 5 deaths. Two of the schizophrenic deaths and one of the affective were due to suicide. The remaining causes of death were distributed across the vascular, respiratory, and malignancy categories. From this study, we are reminded again that the most specific psychiatric diagnosis predictive of premature death is any in the category "organic mental syndrome." These authors found one more demographic factor in their data that was highly predictive of subsequent premature death: age. There was a tenfold higher 4-year mortality among psychiatric patients over 65 compared with those under 59 years.

It is difficult in reviewing all of these data to reach firm conclusions. We prefer the tentative conclusion, not substantiated in every study, that psychiatric patients as a group experience excessive rates of premature death attributable to general medical and neurologic diseases. Older psychiatric patients and psychiatric patients with "organic mental" diagnoses are especially high-risk groups, probably because they are selected for the presence of medical illness. There have not, as yet, been identified specific diagnostic links between major psychiatric diagnoses and major categories of medical illness. The true reasons for this excess mortality among psychiatric patients are not known, but our working presumption in the preparation of this book is that medical problems among psychiatric patients tend to be identified later and treated less effectively than similar problems among other patients. We hope that the chapters that follow will assist psychiatrists in more efficiently and accurately identifying occult general medical illness among their patients.

## PSYCHIATRIC RESPONSIBILITY FOR PHYSICAL ILLNESS

*Clinical Rule No. 2.2*: If the psychiatrist does not identify the medical problems of his or her patients, someone else might, . . . but don't count on it.

We have noticed a curious phenomenon among our psychiatric and general medical colleagues. It seems to us that psychiatrists feel worse about "missing" a general medical or neurologic problem among their patients than do their counterparts in general medicine or surgery when they overlook an emotional disorder. Not everyone might agree with this observation, and there are certainly exceptions among practitioners, but we retain the clear impression that emotional responses differ among specialties with regard to "misses." Typically a psychiatrist feels mortified when he or she discovers that an affective disorder under treatment can be attributed to a brain tumor. An internist who "chases" psychosomatic complaints attributable to an affective disorder is more likely to feel mild annoyance or no particular emotional response.

There are perhaps many dynamic explanations for this phenomenon (assuming that it is at least partly true). We would emphasize two such explanations. First, such an emotional response on the part of the psychiatrist clearly indicates that he or she already feels some *responsibility* for the physical dimension of the patient. In this sense, it is pointless to argue whether psychiatrists *should* feel responsible for medical aspects of their patients—they already do!

Our second dynamic interpretation of psychiatric emotional responses to medical "misses" is a bit more speculative. We have been impressed that the degree of discomfort and embarrassment that appears at least occasionally in the setting of medical misses indicates *guilt* on the part of psychiatrists for not having been more actively involved in the physical assessment or treatment of their patients. Some might contend that this statement represents a projection on our part—which point we will not discuss further. Our interpretation might help in understanding certain contradictions in present-day psychiatric practice. At a time when it has become fashionable to speak of the "biopsychosocial model" in psychiatric practice, very few psychiatrists examine the biological portion of their patients (McIntyre and Romano, 1977; Patterson, 1978). At a time when it is known that patients referred to psychiatry arrive with a liberal mix of undiagnosed or untreated medical problems, psychiatrists in general continue to rely on the theoretically dubious process of "medical clearance" (Weissberg, 1979). Despite a series of papers in recent years advocating that psychiatry receive "primary care" status, we know of no reimbursement system that has done so (Oken and Fink, 1976; Fink, 1977).

Another way of looking at this issue of psychiatric responsibility for the physical status of patients is to consider legal case law which is beginning to emerge in this area (Busch and Cavanaugh, 1985). Although few decisions are yet available, there are cases that have found psychiatrists negligent by reason of an inadequate physical examination or by a failure carefully to review the medical history. It is possible that the courts will construe the medical training of psychiatrists more seriously than do some practitioners and will increasingly hold them responsible for some general medical evaluation of their patients.

This book is designed for those psychiatrists who may wish to begin or to improve their general medical and neurological evaluation skills.

## REFERENCES

Barnes, R. F., Mason, J. C., Greer, C., and Ray, F. T. Medical illness in chronic psychiatric outpatients. *Gen. Hosp. Psychiatry*, 1983, **5**, 191–195.

Browning, C. H., Miller, S. I., and Tyson, R. L. The psychiatric emergency: A high risk medical patient. *Comp. Psychiatry*, 1974, **15**, 153–156.

Bunce, D. F. M., Jones, L. R., Badger, L. W., and Jones, S. E. Medical illness in psychiatric patients: Barriers to diagnosis and treatment. *South. Med. J.*, 1982, **75**, 941–944.

Busch, K. A., and Cavanaugh, J. L. Jr. Physical examination of psychiatric outpatients: Medical and legal issues. *Hosp. Community Psychiatry*, 1985, **36**, 958–961.

Comroe, B. I. Follow-up study of 100 patients diagnosed as "neurosis." *J. Nerv. Ment. Dis.*, 1936, **83**, 679–684.

Dvoredsky, A. E., and Cooley, H. W. Comparative severity of illness in patients with combined medical and psychiatric diagnoses. *Psychosomatics*, 1986, **27**, 625–630.

Eastwood, M. R. *The Relation between Physical and Mental Illness.*, Toronto: University of Toronto Press, 1975.

Eastwood, M. R., Stiasny, S., Meier, H. M. R., and Woogh, C. M. Mental illness and mortality. *Compr. Psychiatry*, 1982, **23**, 377–385.

Fink, P. J. The relationship of psychiatry to primary care. *Am. J. Psychiatry*, 1977, **134**, 126–129.

Hall, R. C. W., Popkin, M. K., Devaul, R. A., Faillace, L. A., and Stickney, S. K. Physical illness presenting as psychiatric disease. *Arch. Gen. Psychiatry*, 1978, **35**, 1315–1320.

Hall, R. C. W., Gardner, E. R., Stickney, S. K., LeCann, A. F., and Popkin, M. K. Physical illness manifesting as psychiatric disease. *Arch. Gen. Psychiatry*, 1980, **37**, 989–995.

Hoenig, J., and Hamilton, M. W. Mortality of psychiatric patients. *Acta Psychiatr. Scand.*, 1966, **42**, 349–361.

Hoffman, R. S. Diagnostic errors in the evaluation of behavioral disorders. *JAMA*, 1982, **248**, 964–967.

Kendler, K. S. A twin study of mortality in schizophrenia and neurosis. *Arch. Gen. Psychiatry*, 1986, **43**, 643–649.

Koranyi, E. K. Fatalities in 2070 psychiatric outpatients. *Arch. Gen. Psychiatry*, 1977, **34**, 1137–1142.

Koranyi, E. K. Morbidity and rate of undiagnosed physical illnesses in a psychiatric clinic population. *Arch. Gen. Psychiatry*, 1979, **36**, 414–419.

Koranyi, E. K. (ed.). *Physical Illness in the Psychiatric Patient*. Springfield, IL: Charles C. Thomas, 1982.

Lipowski, Z. J. Psychiatry of somatic diseases: Epidemiology, pathogenesis, classification. *Compr. Psychiatry*, 1975, **16**, 105–124.

Martin, R. L., Cloninger, C. R., Guze, S. B., and Clayton, P. J. Mortality in a follow-up of 500 psychiatric outpatients. I. Total mortality. *Arch. Gen. Psychiatry*, 1985a, **42**, 47–54.

Martin, R. L., Cloninger, C.R., Guze, S. B., and Clayton, P. J. Mortality in a follow-up of 500 psychiatric outpatients. II. Cause-specific mortality. *Arch. Gen. Psychiatry*, 1985b, **42**, 58–66.

McCarrick, A. K., Manderscheid, R. W., Bertolucci, D. E., Goldman, H., and Tessler, R. C. Chronic medical problems in the chronically mentally ill. *Hosp. Community Psychiatry*, 1986, **37**, 289–291.

McIntyre, J. S., and Romano, J. Is there a stethoscope in the house (and is it used)? *Arch. Gen. Psychiatry*, 1977, **34**, 1147–1151.

Murphy, J. M., Monson, R. R., Olivier, D. C., Sobol, A. M., and Leighton, A. H. Affective disorders and mortality: A general population study. *Arch. Gen. Psychiatry*, 1987, **44**, 473–480.

Oken, D., and Fink, P. J. General psychiatry: A primary-care specialty. *JAMA*, 1976, **235**, 1973–1974.

Patterson, C. W. Psychiatrists and physical examinations: A survey. *Am. J. Psychiatry*, 1978, **135**, 967–968.

Rorsman, B., Hagnell, O., and Lanke, J. Mortality in the Lundby study: Natural death in different forms of mental disorder in a total population investigated during a 25-year period. *Neuropsychobiology*, 1982, **8**, 188–197.

Singer, E., Garfinkel, R., Cohen, S. M., and Srole, L. Mortality and mental health: Evidence from the Midtown Manhattan restudy. *Soc. Sci. Med.*, 1976, **10**, 517–525.

Tsuang, M. T., Woolson, R. F., and Fleming, J. A. Causes of death in schizophrenia and manic-depression. *Br. J. Psychiatry*, 1980, **136**, 239–242.

Weissberg, M. P. Emergency room medical clearance: An educational problem. *Am. J. Psychiatry*, 1979, **136**, 787–790.

Winokur, G., and Block, D. W. Psychiatric and medical diagnoses as risk factors for mortality in psychiatric patients: A case-control study. *Am. J. Psychiatry*, 1987, **144**, 208–211.

Wynne-Davies, D. General medical problems in a psychiatric hospital. *Lancet*, 1964, **i**, 545–548.

Wynne-Davies, D. Physical illness in psychiatric outpatients. *Br. J. Psychiatry*, 1965, **111**, 27–33.

# 3

# The Neurological Examination

Our presentation in this chapter of a general outline by which one might approach the neurologic examination is somewhat artificial in that the examination is discussed in isolation from the neurologic history. In practice, history and examination are dynamically related. One gets a sense from the clinical history of what *might* be wrong, and the hierarchy of these possibilities is then measured against the examination. After the examination, the "odds ratios" for various structural and functional abnormalities of the nervous system are adjusted, and further diagnostic testing is selected or postponed. We have chosen to focus this chapter on the examination as opposed to the clinical history and interview, because psychiatric clinicians are usually excellent at the latter and clumsy at the former. We have not forgotten, however, that the clinical history directs and focuses the examination, and salient historical issues are discussed in the separate chapters with the various disease syndromes.

---

*Clinical Rule 3.1*: If you must see a new patient in 30 min, take the history for 29 min and examine for 1.

---

Although the neurological examination is always influenced by the clinical history, there is still a structure to the examination that cannot be ignored. The tendon stretch reflexes are always checked at least cursorily, but with greater care when the patient complains of focal weakness. In this sense, there is always a balance between an individual clinician's "standard" examination and the examination that fits a particular patient. The balance probably differs for each clinician, and this is fine. We do not agree entirely with Anderson (1980), who suggested that psychiatrists might determine their physical observations by their mental status findings. This is partly true but fails to take account of the autonomous structure of both general medical and neurologic examinations.

We are disappointed when psychiatrists object to performing physical and neurological examinations on the grounds that they cannot do the examination thoroughly and accurately. Because of their skills and experience in interview and mental-status assessments, psychiatric clinicians have an important advantage in the neurological examination of their patients. We know that when psychiatrists begin to examine their patients, physical illnesses are identified (Summers *et al.*, 1981). With time, experience, and repetition, the physical examinations become individualized within each practitioner's diagnostic and therapeutic repertoire. Fewer coexisting medical syndromes are overlooked, and greater diagnostic certainty develops. The most difficult physical examination for the clinical psychiatrist is the *first* one.

There are two additional points that deserve emphasis with regard to the neurologic examination. Clinicians have available to them a growing arsenal of neurodiagnostic laboratory and imaging tests. All are expensive. All require clinical judgment for effective use. Psychiatrists share rightly in the gatekeeping function for this neurodiagnostic arsenal. The neurologic examination, for example, can assist in avoiding the appearance of an unending series of normal head CT scan reports in psychiatric patients' charts (Larson *et al.*, 1981; Beresford *et al.*, 1985). The examination not only assists the clinician in selecting which line of neurodiagnostic testing to pursue, but it helps in deciding how aggressive to be in pursuing tests and consultations.

Two other general comments should be made concerning the neurological examination and psychiatric patients. The first is that psychiatric patients in general demonstrate abnormalities on the neurological examination that seem to be related to the psychiatric disease itself (Woods *et al.*, 1986; Tucker *et al.*, 1975; Mukherjee *et al.*, 1984). In patients with affective disorders, such findings may be attributable to psychotropic medications, but in schizophrenic patients, no obvious explanation for the finding is apparent. The findings are not always "soft" or nonlocalizing, but may implicate oculomotor or motor systems and may be asymmetric. In the study by Woods and colleagues, blinded neurologic examiners found that 19 of 24 schizophrenic patients had at least one neurologic finding from the list presented in Table 3.1.

And lastly, it should be admitted that the neurological examination we present in this chapter is in no sense a complete one. Some might object that it is not even a *thorough* one, to which we would respond that a thorough description of the neurological examination would require a book in itself. Several such books have appeared in recent years (DeJong, 1979; Wells and Duncan, 1980; Mancall, 1981; Wiederholt, 1982; Van Allen and Rodnitzky, 1981), and the interested reader is referred to them. We hope to describe an outline approach to the examination, emphasizing functional assessment of the various neurological systems. This examination derives from that which we use and teach within the Departments of Psychiatry and Neurology at the University of Rochester.

**Table 3.1**
Overview Neurologic Examination[a]

| Sign number | Description |
|---|---|
| 1 | Dementia |
| 2 | Acute delirium/confusion |
| 3 | Aphasia |
| 4 | Ophthalmoplegia (specify type) |
| 5 | Anosmia |
| 6–7 | Esophoria [right (R) eye, left (L) eye] |
| 8–9 | Exophoria (R eye, L eye) |
| 10 | Gaze nystagmus |
| 11–12 | Facial weakness (R, L) |
| 13–14 | Hearing loss (R ear, L ear) |
| 15 | Dysarthria |
| 16 | Buccolingual dyskinesia |
| 17–22 | Sensory loss, central |
| | Face (R, L) |
| | Arm (R, L) |
| | Leg (R, L) |
| 23–26 | Motor weakness, central |
| | Arm/hand (R, L) |
| | Leg (R, L) |
| 27–30 | Motor weakness, peripheral |
| | Arm/hand (R, L) |
| | Leg (R, L) |
| 31–34 | Spastic rigidity |
| | Arm (R, L) |
| | Leg (R, L) |
| 35–38 | Cogwheel rigidity |
| | Arm (R, L) |
| | Leg (R, L) |
| 39–42 | Hypotonia |
| | Arm (R, L) |
| | Leg (R, L) |
| 43–47 | Postural (toxic/metabolic) tremor |
| | Head |
| | Arm (R, L) |
| | Leg (R, L) |
| 48–52 | Resting tremor |
| | Head |
| | Hand (R, L) |
| | Foot (R, L) |
| 53–54 | Intention tremor |
| | Hand (R, L) |
| 55–56 | Choreiform movements |
| | Hand (R, L) |
| 57–58 | Slow/clumsy alternating movements |
| 59–60 | Mirror movements |
| | Hand (R, L) |

*(continued)*

Table 3.1 *(Continued)*

| Sign number | Description |
|---|---|
| 61 | Whole-body akinesia |
| 62 | Whole-body clumsiness |
| 63 | Balance abnormality |
| 64 | Gait ataxia |
| 65 | Parkinsonian gait |
| | Reflex hyperactivity |
| | Arm (R, L) |
| | Knee (R, L) |
| 66–71 | Ankle (R, L) |
| 72–73 | Babinski's sign (R, L) |
| 74–75 | Grasp reflex (R, L) |
| 76–77 | Pes cavus (R, L) |
| 78 | Mild cognitive impairment/mental retardation |
| 79 | Other |

[a]From Woods *et al.* (1986).

## MENTAL STATUS

A good interview produces reliable observations for the most important section of the neurologic examination, the mental status. Psychiatrists have a great advantage over other physicians during this portion of the examination because of their training and experience with the medical interview. A great number of mental status observations may potentially be made during any interview. What follows is an outline of mental status categories, organized hierarchically within the neuraxis, which we have found applicable to patients across a wide spectrum of clinical conditions. For more detailed discussion of mental status assessment, the reader is referred to several recent texts (Strub and Black, 1985; Mesulam, 1985; Cummings, 1985).

### Consciousness

We consider that there are two dimensions to consciousness as a mental function, each with its own neurologic implication. If one considers mental life as playing upon the stage of consciousness, there are two separate lighting systems—the klieg lights and the spotlights. The klieg lights provide diffuse illumination for the stage, analogous to the diffuse quality of arousal, alertness, or "with-it-ness." This diffuse background arousal quality of consciousness is supported by that set of diffuse, ascending brainstem tegmental systems which we group under the heading "reticular activating system" (Plum and Posner,

1980). This quality of consciousness is probably most closely correlated with general EEG background rate.

Good clinicians intuitively assess the arousal dimension of consciousness first, because if the patient has a problem with consciousness, the examiner has got a problem. Although certain manic and depressed states may in themselves account for alteration of consciousness, by far the majority of such conditions are metabolic or neurologic in etiology. Immediately upon making an observation of impaired consciousness, the examiner shifts his diagnostic agenda toward identifying a treatable medical or neurologic disease. The remainder of the mental status examination is of dubious validity in such circumstances anyway and may properly be abbreviated after careful observations concerning consciousness have been documented.

Remembering that arousal dysfunction is a spectrum disorder, ranging from coma to diffusely hyperalert states, the examiner merely records observations during a series of systematic interventions:

| | |
|---|---|
| Baseline arousal description | Does the patient spontaneously look at the examiner? Is there evidence for hyperalertness? Are his eyes open? |
| Arousal to voice | With language addressed to the patient, what happens? Do his eyes open? Does he look at the examiner? |
| Arousal to shake | With physical touching, what happens? Does the patient wake up? What does he do? |
| Arousal to pain | With painful stimulation, what is the patient's response? |

*Note*: The administration of painful stimulation to a patient is not the time for flamboyance or for unusual creativity. Pinching the first dorsal interosseous muscle or rolling a pencil against the base of a fingernail is quite sufficient.

What we have termed the "spotlight" quality of consciousness refers to the complex ability to focus one's attention on a particular stimulus or task and to maintain the focus for a period of time. The neuroanatomy of focused and maintained attention is more hemispheric and cortical than that of arousal. Normal "attentional" function probably requires intact prefrontal cortex, parietal cortex, and subcortical relays in cingulum and basal ganglia (Mesulam, 1981). In right-handed people, the right hemisphere is dominant for attention maintenance (Denes *et al.*, 1982), and lesions of that hemisphere produce more severe inattention syndromes than do lesions of the left hemisphere. While the arousal quality of consciousness is most often impaired by diffuse toxic or metabolic conditions, this attention-focusing ability is most often impaired by focal structural disease of one or both cerebral hemispheres. Typically, these patients are normally alert, but they are distractable, often tangential, and difficult to engage. Mental status tests that require continuous performance by the patient are the best indices of general arousal.

## Serial Digit Repetition

The patient is asked to repeat a series of random digits after the examiner has presented each list. The digits are given at 1-sec intervals, and the patient's response is recorded. After the patient's limit in forward repetition has been determined, the process is repeated asking him to reverse the digit order.

7 3
2 9 1
6 2 7 4
8 1 3 5 2 "Patient cannot do—reverses last two digits."

6 5
1 7 8 "Patient cannot do—reverts to forward repetition."

These criteria for a "normal" performance on this task are more a function of the examiner's judgment than any of us would like to admit. However, as a general rule, outpatients of average intelligence can repeat seven digits forward and reverse five. Inpatients on any service do well to repeat five forward and three in reverse.

## Serial Subtractions

We have yet to encounter a physician who can satisfactorily explain this task in less than 5 min to a naive inpatient. A more efficient approach is as follows:

*Physician*: "Please subtract 7 from 100."
*Patient*: "93."
*Physician*: "Now subtract 7 from 93."
*Patient*: "86."
*Physician*: "Continue that way until zero."

It is always worthwhile to write down the patient's responses just as he produces them. The evaluation of his performance as normal or abnormal is a separate matter from the observations of his performance and should be entered in a different area of the write-up. In general, two errors represent the limit of normal performance in this task. Unfortunately, most of these tasks are partly a function of education. For patients who have not completed high school, subtraction of serial 3's may be substituted. Serial 1's (essentially counting backward from 100) may also be used.

Mental status tests that may be more specifically related to the frontal lobe regulation of attention include the following:

### Serial Word List Generation

The patient is asked to generate a list of words from a conceptual category (animals) or beginning with a certain letter during a 60-sec time period. The number of responses is counted. Typically, 10–14 responses per category can be expected during a 60-sec interval (Lezak, 1983).

### Alternating Sequences Test

Susceptibility to interference can be assessed by asking the patient to produce a continuous line of "m's" and "n's" across a page without lifting his pencil from the page (Luria, 1966). Patients who cannot inhibit competing responses are unable to do this.

## Language

After consciousness, the examiner considers the patient's language. Both of these mental functions are "enabling" in the sense that impairments can render invalid the testing of subsequent mental status functions. Anyone who has attempted to obtain a clinical history from an aphasic patient can understand this statement. When an aphasia is suspected, it is wise to turn the examination directly to an assessment of language function.

We are much indebted to the late Norman Geschwind and his colleagues for their investigations of the interconnections between left cerebral hemispheric structures and language function (Geschwind, 1971). The following bedside language examination presents an outline for approaching this mental status function. For initial clinical encounters, a practical goal for the examiner is to obtain some information about each of the following six language functions:

1. Fluency. Fluency refers to the rhythm and "flow" of the patient's speech. Does the patient have the ability to produce spontaneous speech without unusual prompting? Are words produced at a normal rate? Are paraphasic errors made? Are helping words and modifying words appropriately interposed? This judgment of fluent versus nonfluent aphasia types sounds simple but requires clinical experience to become reliable.
2. Naming. Can the patient name a watch and its four principal compo-

nents (face or dial, stem, band, clasp)? His performance may be scored accordingly (i.e., "names four of five watch parts").

3. Comprehension. Does the patient follow a one-stage command? How often? How about two-stage commands? Can he read a narrative paragraph (standardized to each examiner's clinical experience) and understand it? Example:

*Examiner*: "Stick out your tongue," or "Close your eyes."

A command that involves crossing the midline, or concepts of left and right is more difficult:

*Examiner*: "Show me your left hand."
"Place your right hand on your left ear."

In testing verbal comprehension, the examiner should avoid giving nonverbal clues, many of which have become second nature in common discourse.

4. Repetition. Can the patient repeat a phrase of one-syllable words (the most difficult repetition task): "No ifs, ands, or buts." Can the patient repeat a single word?
5. Reading. Can the patient read the narrative paragraph aloud?
6. Writing. Can the patient write a sentence (save this as written in the chart)?

For the examiner, what counts is not the mellifluousness of the observations but their accuracy. With some data for each of these six language functions, an initial aphasia classification can be made at the bedside (Fig. 3.1). The reader can see that reasonable accuracy in bedside aphasia judgments depends on pattern recognition. The aphasia subtypes are not distinguished by total impairment of *this* language function juxtaposed to fully normal performance in *that* one, but rather by a preponderant dysfunction here as opposed to there. The reader may take heart, however. The human brain is not as good as the IBM PC at registering bits of information (see following section), but it is probably much better than the machine at recognizing patterns in human behavior.

## Memory, Verbal and Visual

Papez (1937) thought that the limbic circuit involving hippocampus–fornix–mamillary body–dorsal nucleus of the thalamus was the neuroanatomic system, which subserves the "stream of emotion." It might be more accurate to say that these structures subserve the "stream of memory." Current neuroscientific investigations indicate a major role for mesial temporal, posterior hypothalamic, and dorsal thalamic structures in memory function (Lynch *et al.*, 1984).

| Fluent aphasia? | | Nonfluent aphasia? | |
|---|---|---|---|
| Comprehension poor<br>Repetition poor<br>Reading poor<br>↓<br>*Wernicke's-type aphasia*<br>Anatomy of lesion involves posterior portion of superior temporal gyrus, left hemisphere; portions of inferior parietal lobule often involved | Comprehension poor<br>Repetition not bad<br>Reading not bad<br>↓<br>*Transcortical sensory-type aphasia*<br>Anatomy of lesion involves parietal language association areas, sparing Wernicke's area itself | Comprehension not bad<br>Repetition poor<br>Reading not bad<br>↓<br>*Broca's-type aphasia*<br>Anatomy of lesion involves posterior area of third frontal gyrus, left hemisphere | Comprehension not bad<br>Repetition not bad<br>Reading not bad<br>↓<br>*Transcortical motor-type aphasia*<br>Anatomy of lesion may involve anterior portion of internal capsule |
| Comprehension not bad<br>Repetition poor<br>Reading not bad<br>↓<br>*Conduction-type aphasia*<br>Anatomy of lesion involves arcuate fasciculus, left hemisphere. | | | |

**Figure 3.1.** Classification of aphasia.

In this outline, we present a bedside approach to the testing of verbal and visual memory. This approach is brief and suitable for those who must make clinical decisions. It is one of many possible approaches, and it is not exhaustive. We believe it is important to test and record visual memory function separately from verbal memory function, because there is some evidence of hemispheric specialization in these functions (left hemisphere—verbal; right hemisphere—visuospatial).

## Verbal Memory

### Three-Word Test.

There is nothing wrong with the three-word verbal memory used almost universally by practicing neurologists. It is brief and practical, and it provides some limited objective information concerning the patient's verbal learning ability. It is administered as follows:

*Physician:* "I am going to tell you a list of three objects and ask you to remember them. Are you ready?"
*Patient:* "Ready."
*Physician:* "White rose, Cadillac, Portland Avenue. Now say them back so I know you have got them."
*Patient:* "White rose, Cadillac, Portland Avenue."

Five minutes later, after interposition of a subsequent mental status test:

*Physician:* "Can you tell me those three objects I asked you to remember?"
*Patient:* "White rose . . ."
*Physician:* "One was a motor car."
*Patient:* "Cadillac."
*Physician:* "One began with the sound Pah . . ."
*Patient:* "Portland Avenue."

The clinical value of this test can be increased by recording carefully the patient's responses ("learns three complex objects in a single trial; recalls one of them at 5 min spontaneously; three with phonemic and categorical cues") and providing phonemic and categorical cues for missed items. A person with normal memory function should make no errors on this test.

### Ten-Word List.

A more formalized and expanded version of the three-object test will provide a more sensitive measure of memory function (Table 3.2). Here the examiner presents the patient with a list of ten words (no place names or proper nouns), spaced verbally at 1-sec intervals. The patient is asked to repeat the entire list after each trial, and his responses are recorded until the list is repeated once correctly. The order of his responses should be indicated by numbers.

The patient can be asked for spontaneous recall of the words after 5 min of distraction (active recall) and can be asked to select the words from a list of

**Table 3.2**
Ten-Word List to Test Memory Function

| Word list | Trial 1 | Trial 2 | Trial 3 | Trial 4 |
|---|---|---|---|---|
| Yellow | 1 | 1 | 1 | 1 |
| Erase | 2 | 2 | 2 | 2 |
| Lake | | 3 | | 3 |
| Confers | | | | 4 |
| Apple | | | 6 | 5 |
| Quickly | | | 7 | 6 |
| Compound | | | | 7 |
| Purchase | | 4 | 3 | 8 |
| Woolen | 3 | 5 | 4 | 9 |
| Auto | 4 | 6 | 5 | 10 |

20 distractors (recognition recall). The test is not easy to perform correctly, but persons of average intelligence or above and in no major distress should be able to repeat the list in four trials. A normal strategy is for the patient to "close in" the list from both ends, as illustrated.

### Visuoconstructive Skills and Visual Memory

There are many tests that measure aspects of these mental functions. One relatively simple but reliable way is for the physician to present the patient with a complex geometric figure (laminated and standardized to the experience of the individual examiner) for a period of 10 sec. The figure is removed, and the patient is asked to reproduce it (immediate visual recall). The figure is then returned to the patient, and he is asked to copy it (visual copy). After 5 min of distraction, the patient is asked to reproduce the figure from memory (delayed visual recall). A sample figure might be as shown in Fig. 3.2, although clinicians can make their own.

## Emotional State

It would not be appropriate for us in this book to discuss the assessment of the emotional state by psychiatric clinicians. The interested reader is referred

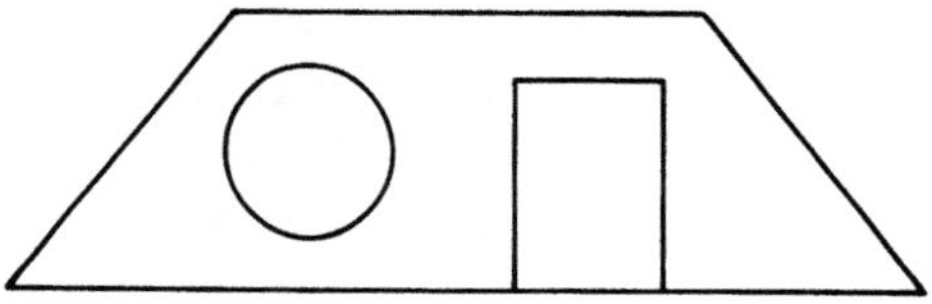

**Figure 3.2.** A sample test for visual memory.

to one of several recent texts on psychiatric interviewing (Reiser and Schroder, 1980). We would mention only one caveat for the examiner with regard to emotional assessment. Whenever the possibility of structural or metabolic neurologic disease arises, it is worth remembering that the neurologic systems that subserve expressed affect ("affective display") differ from those systems that subserve the subjective, experienced side of an emotion ("affective sensation"). Occasionally, these systems are selectively involved by a neuropathological process (Schiffer *et al.*, 1985), such as in the syndrome of pathological laughing and weeping.

### Personality

We do not discuss methods of assessment during interview in this book. This in no way diminishes the importance of this dimension of the mental status. The reader is again referred to the texts concerning psychiatric interviewing.

### Abstractions, Similarities, Fund of Knowledge, Metaphors, and Proverbs

There is a vast array of mental status tests to assess these functions, which are sometimes designated "higher cognitive functions." These assessments are not typically part of bedside mental status assessments but are more likely to be part of more comprehensive neuropsychological batteries. It is probably safe to say that we know less concerning the neurologic systems subserving these functions than we do about the functional areas described earlier. Again, the interested reader is referred to textbooks for more information.

## CRANIAL NERVES

In this outline approach to cranial nerve examination, we have continued to sacrifice obsessive completeness for what we hope will be functional utility. The neuroanatomy of the cranial nerves is more complex than that of any other examination portion. The precise interpretation of neuropathologic findings may well require referral to one of the neurologic examination texts cited above or to a textbook of neurology (see, e.g., Baker and Joynt, 1986; Adams and Victor, 1985; Rowland, 1984)). Ironically, however, it is probably easier to recognize that something is wrong with the cranial nerves than with other portions of the nervous system, if one has even a minimal functional approach to the examination. We will outline such an approach.

## Cranial Nerve 1 (Olfactory Nerve)

The testing of this cranial nerve in psychiatric patients yields too many false-positive results to be of clinical use.

## Cranial Nerves 2, 3, 4, 6 (Optic, Oculomotor, Trochlear, and Abducens Nerves)

We group these four cranial nerves together, because they all have to do with the function of the eye, its acuity, and its movements. We recommend the following initial examination.

### Acuity

Check acuity first. It is alarming to see how often the testing of this, the primary ocular function, is omitted. Since we are interested in function over refraction, the patient is encouraged to wear prescribed corrective lenses. Test each eye separately. The easiest instrument to use is a laminated Jaeger Card (Fig. 3.3), which can be purchased at most medical bookstores. The card should be held 14 inches from the patient's eye. Record the smallest line read correctly with two or fewer errors ("acuity $J_2$ minus 1").

### Visual Fields

Visual field cuts and scotomata vary in size and density as a function of the target presented. One must always record, for example, that the visual fields are normal or abnormal to a specific target. A small object of red color, such as a match head, is more sensitive to field defects than is a larger white object or a white light. The standard confrontation test object, a wiggling finger, is the least sensitive test object. The examiner can easily place two matches in his bag to be used for assessing visual fields.

The examiner sits facing the patient, at a face-to-face distance of 18–20 inches. The patient is asked to close one eye and to stare at the pupil of the examiner's corresponding eye. The examiner closes his opposite eye and fixes gaze upon the patient's open eye. The visual-field targets are brought by the examiner from outside the mutual visual perimeter toward the midline, as indicated in Fig. 3.4. Each eye is tested separately, and defects are recorded. For example, "left homonymous hemianopsia to 3-mm red target."

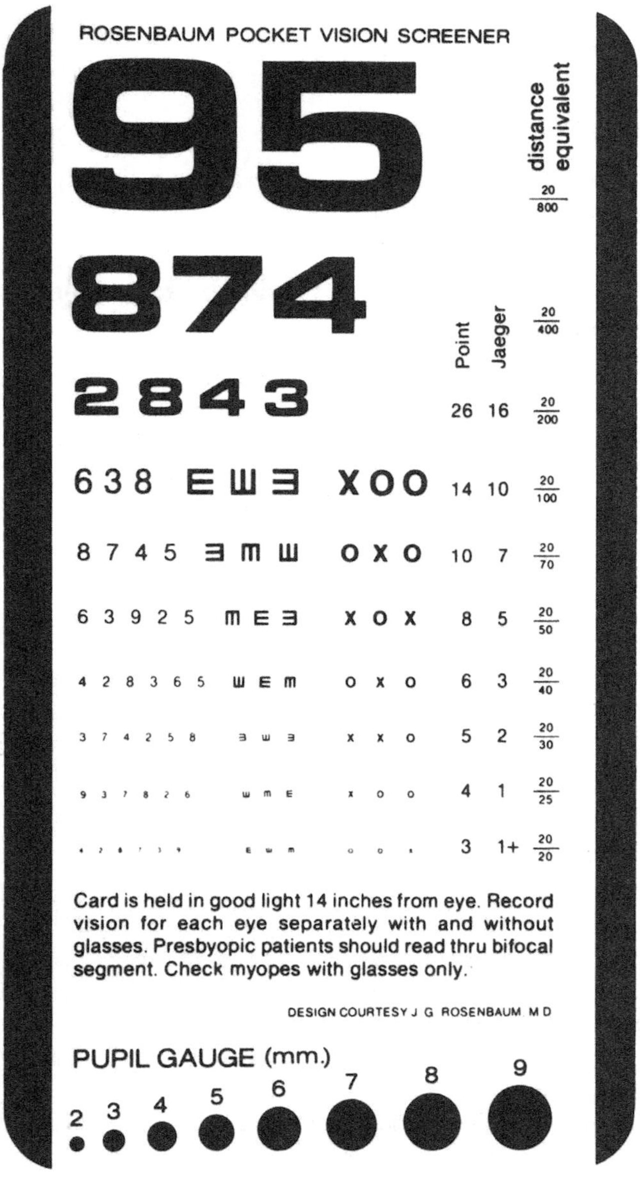


**Figure 3.3.** Laminated Jaeger Card tests visual acuity.

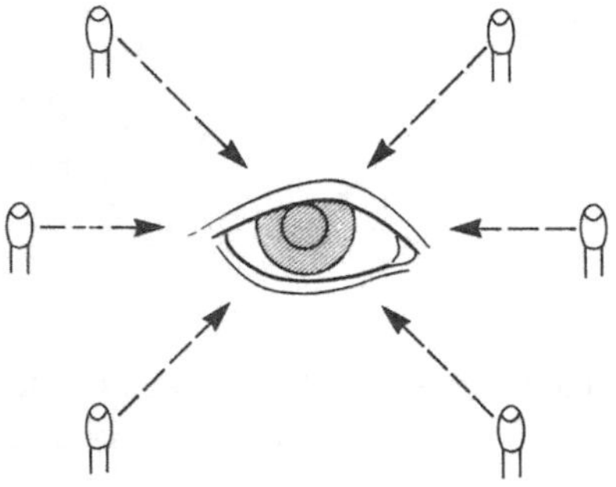

**Figure 3.4.** Visual-field testing by method of confrontation.

## Pupillary Light Response

All reflexes are more complex in their neural circuitry than we would like to think. The pupillary constriction response to bright light requires an afferent mechanism (optic nerve), an effector mechanism (oculomotor nerve), and coordinating connections between the two. The examiner should develop experience with this reflex under controlled conditions. The room should be darkened, including shades, for a few moments while the light is assembled. A bright light should be used, such as the tubular fiber optic attachment that may be purchased for the opthalmoscope. Do not substitute the 89¢ lights that the bookstore sells! Each pupil should first be tested directly, and then the consensual response should be noted. Develop a "feel" for the normal speed of the constriction, which should be quite brisk. Remember that 15–20% of people may normally have a 1-mm asymmetry in pupil size prior to constriction.

## Funduscopy

While the room remains darkened, the patient is asked to fixate on a distant spot to immobilize the eyes, and the optic discs, retina, and vasculature are examined. This is difficult to do well with psychiatric patients. What is reasonable to expect, however, is for the examiner to develop familiarity with the range of normal findings over time, so that the occasional papilledema, hemorrhage, or retinitis will be recognized. Again, it is more important to recognize that something might be wrong than to know what it is. More extensive texts may be read (Miller, 1982), but experience teaches best.

## Eye Movements

The extraocular muscles are innervated by cranial nerves 3 (medial rectus, superior rectus, inferior rectus, inferior oblique), 4 (superior oblique), and 6

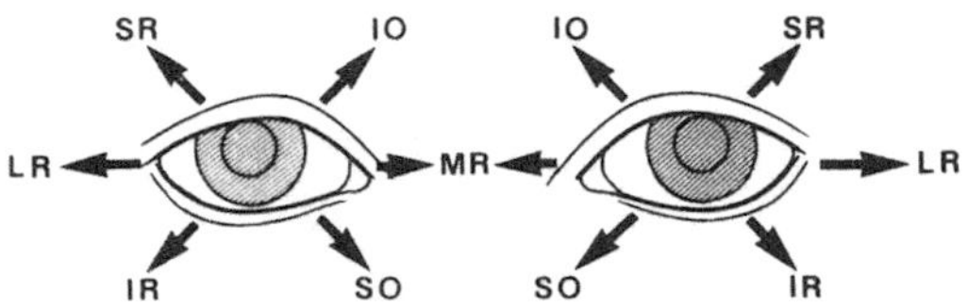


**Figure 3.5.** Primary actions of extraoculor muscles. LR, lateral rectus; MR, medial rectus; SR, superior rectus; IR, inferior rectus; SO, superior oblique; IO, inferior oblique.

(lateral rectus). Specific extraocular muscles are maximally engaged when the patient's eyes move to the following positions as seen by the examiner (Fig. 3.5).

One can elicit more information from this examination by remembering that there are several different systems within the neuraxis that govern eye movements. Frontal-lobe-mediated systems govern voluntary conjugate movements (saccades); parietal-lobe-mediated systems govern tracking and pursuit movements; and brainstem-located cerebellar and vestibular systems govern postural gaze reflexes (oculocephalic responses). The examiner sits facing the patient as for testing visual fields and notes any strabismus in direct forward gaze. The patient is then asked to sweep his gaze successively "way to the left," then "way to the right," then "way up," then "way down." After these voluntary movements are tested, pursuit of a target such as the examiner's finger into these same fields of gaze is tested. Subjective diplopia is sought, and nystagmus or extraocular palsies are noted.

Subtle abnormalities of eye movements, such as a unilateral extraocular muscle weakness on lateral gaze, are best appreciated when the examiner fixes his gaze not on the patient's eyes but on a midpoint at the bridge of the patient's nose.

## Cranial Nerves 5 and 7 (Trigeminal and Facial)

These two nerves are grouped functionally and in assessment, since they provide sensory and motor innervation to face and jaw. Can the patient chew? Can the patient feel his face? Can the patient move his face? The separate muscles innervated by these two cranial nerves are listed in Table 3.3, and the topography of the three sensory dimensions of the trigeminal nerve are depicted in Figure 3.6.

### Mastication

When the motor division of cranial nerve 5 is impaired, the patient demonstrates weakness in raising, depressing, protruding, retracting, and deviating the mandible. The mandible moves *toward* the weak side in trigeminal paralysis, and the patient has difficulty moving it with strength toward the normally

**Table 3.3**
Orofacial Muscles Innervated by Cranial Nerves 5 and 7

| 5 | 7 |
|---|---|
| Temporalis | Orbicularis oculi |
| Masseter | Corrugator |
| Pterygoid | Buccinator |
| Mylohyoid | Orbicularis oris |
| Anterior digastricus | Platysma |
| Tensor veli palatini | Stylohyoid |
| | Posterior digastricus |
| | Stapedius |

innervated side. In conversion disorders, the opposite pattern may be seen. Since the motor nuclei of cranial nerve 5 receive mostly bilateral supranuclear innervation, paresis of these muscles tends to be seen only with pathology of the brainstem or base of skull. Trauma and tumor are the most likely causes.

## Facial Movements and Symmetry

Fortunately or unfortunately, everyone's face demonstrates some left/right asymmetry. This fact is probably of major heuristic significance with regard to the functional differences between the hemispheres, but it is more of a nuisance in judging subtle facial palsies. Again, the examiner should sit facing the patient at equal height and for a few movements just observe carefully. How symmetric is the asymmetry? Emotionally driven asymmetries are more likely

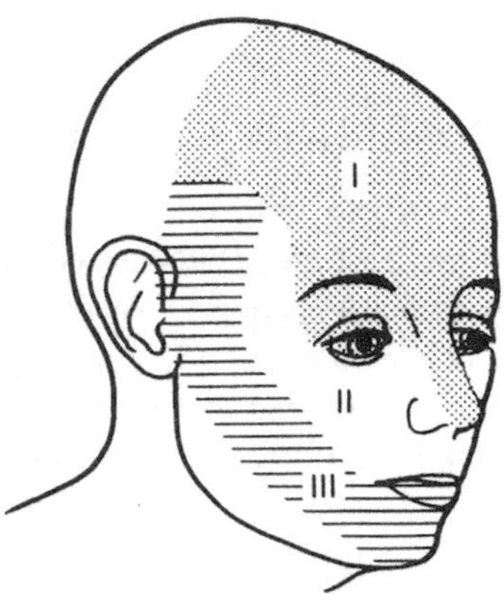


**Figure 3.6.** Sensory divisions of trigeminal nerve.

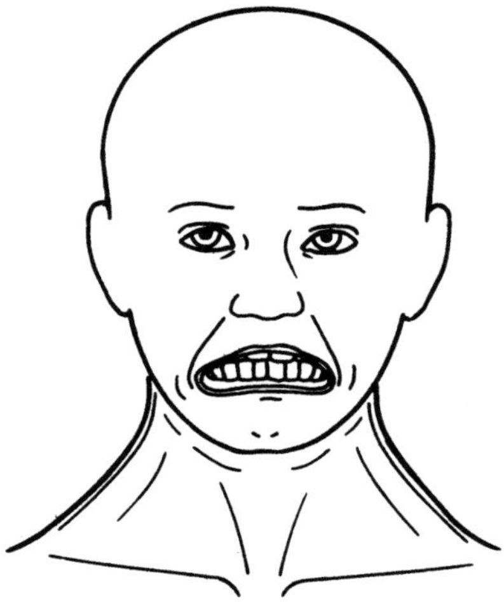

**Figure 3.7.** Tensing of platysma in examination of cranial nerve 7.

to affect the angle of the mouth; upper motor neuron pattern palsies tend to flatten the nasolabial fold on the side of the face opposite the lesion. It is useful to remember that the seventh nerve also innervates platysma in the neck. One can ask the patient to "show your bad face" by tensing the neck (Fig. 3.7), in which case the folds of platysma may actually be counted on left and right sides. In supranuclear weakness of cranial nerve 7 (which is most common among psychiatric patients), the weakness is more apparent in the lower two-thirds of the face, with more symmetric function of forehead musculature.

When abnormalities of facial movement are present, the examiner may wish to tell the patient a joke. Facial movements that relate to emotional states such as mirth are controlled by different neurologic systems from those that have to do with voluntary movements. Some patients with hemispheric cortical lesions may demonstrate upper motor neuron type weakness of cranial nerve 7, yet have normal strength for emotional movements of the face.

## Cranial Nerve 8 (Acoustic)

Along with olfactory and visual acuity, hearing is probably one of the three least frequently tested cranial nerve functions, despite its importance in psychiatric patients. The eighth nerve actually subserves vestibular function along with auditory perception, and the function is not tested very often either. We recommend that the examiner consider these two functions of nerve 8 separately, and routinely test one or two functions from each division of the nerve.

### Conversational Acuity

Does the patient hear and respond to ordinary conversation?

## Whispered Numbers

Auditory perception may be assessed to three individual whispered numbers in each ear. Nonlabial sounds, such as "eight" and "one," may be more difficult to hear. The test is admittedly impossible to standardize across examiners, but it may become reliable with experience for the individual examiner. And the test assesses the most important auditory function—hearing the spoken word (or number).

## Weber Test

The Weber and Rinne tests are of value in distinguishing neurogenic hearing impairments from those due to middle-ear disease. A 256-cps tuning fork should be used (a 512-cps fork is handy for testing higher-frequency perception, but save the 128-cps for peripheral vibratory sensation testing). The fork is struck and placed on the vertex of the skull in the midline, and the patient is asked if it is louder in one ear or about the same in both. The Weber lateralizes *toward* unilateral middle-ear deafness and *away* from unilateral sensorineural deafness.

## Rinne Test

The tuning fork is lightly struck, then placed with its foot against the patient's mastoid process behind the ear (bone conduction). After a few moments for the stimulus to register, the fork is removed, and the vibrating heads are placed 2 inches from the ear (air conduction). The patient is asked which is louder. Bone conduction becomes louder than air conduction in middle-ear disease, but the AC > BC pattern is retained in sensorineural deafness.

## Vestibular Functions

The vestibular apparatus, nerve, and nuclei subserve complicated postural reflexes involving head, eyes, trunk, and limbs. They are mostly unconscious, but can generate sensations of vertigo and spatial disorientation when disturbed. Some testing of vestibular function can be performed at the bedside.

Nystagmus. Many patients with vestibular disease have nystagmus. It is typically conjugate and rhythmic. It may be related to sudden movement of head or neck, or to postural change.

Postural Deviation. Truncal orientation is dependent upon intact vestibular function, although cerebellar and sensory systems are also involved. Patients may be asked to perform the Romberg maneuver; stand with feet touching and eyes closed while maintaining balance. Patients with vestibular damage tend to fall in a persisting direction.

Past-Pointing. On finger-to-nose testing, the patient may be asked to close his eyes while his index finger is alternating from his nose to the examiner's hand. Patients with vestibular lesions tend to gradually deviate in a certain direction.

## Cranial Nerves 9, 10, 11, 12 (Glossopharyngeal, Vagus, Accessory, and Hypoglossal)

We combine these four cranial nerves for testing and recording purposes because of their medullary anatomy. Disease of the medulla is rarely mistaken for psychiatric disease. We recommend a brief, functional approach to these last four cranial nerves as follows:

### Nerves 9 and 10

Both of these nerves have motor efferents to palatal and pharyngeal musculature, as well as autonomic efferents. Posterior pharyngeal sensation and taste are also subserved by the glossopharyngeal nerve. One performs a functional screening examination in listening to the patient's speech. Is there hoarseness or change in voice quality? Elevation of the soft palate can be observed quickly when the mouth is open, and pharyngeal sensation can be tested with a tongue blade (although we do not routinely do this).

### Nerve 11

The spinal accessory and medullary portions of this nerve innervate the trapezius and sternocleidomastoid muscles. Observe the patient carefully at rest and during shoulder shrugging. Is one side lower or slower than the other? Shoulder elevation against resistance may also be tested. Sternocleidomastoid is tested by having the patient laterally rotate the chin against resistance. Remember that the left SCM rotates the chin to the *right*.

### Nerve 12

Tongues are tough. Observations of the tongue are most useful in psychiatric patients as early evidence for movements disorders—dystonias and tardive dyskinesia. Since abnormal movements are most readily seen when the patient does not know he is being observed, the tongue is best studied while the patient is saying "ahhh" and elevating his palate.

## MOTOR SYSTEMS

There are 188 individual muscles in the human body, most of which can be tested in relative isolation and graded for strength using the recommendations of the Medical Research Council (1943): 0, no contraction; 1, trace contraction only; 2, active movement with gravity eliminated; 3, active movement against gravity; 4, weak, but motion against resistance; 5, normal strength.

This approach is rarely useful or reliable within psychiatric patient groups. Functional testing of muscle groups is much more effective, requiring only keen observation by the examiner and a willingness to make judgments about the range of normal. The screening examination that follows is based on the one we use and teach at the University of Rochester. We suggest that it be done in the order outlined.

### Ambulation

Watch the patient walk as unobtrusively as possible. Not only is it polite to have the patient precede you to the examining room, but it also provides the most ingenuous gait observations of the entire examination. Observe *station,* which is the patient's manner of standing with feet approximated. Observe *gait* for weakness, ataxia, or asymmetry. Note any asymmetry of *associated movements.* Subtle hemiparesis may be evident in a *postural* asymmetry, with flexion and internal rotation of the arm matched with extension and external rotation of the leg. Ask the patient to perform tandem walking, heel walking, and toe walking, and record whether he can do it. For a patient on anticonvulsants, the time during which he can balance with feet approximated and eyes closed may be used as an objective measure of toxicity.

### Upper Extremities

The patient should be at least relatively undressed for the remainder of the motor and reflex examination. Observe muscle tone first, by passively flexing and extending the patient's forearms on the elbows. If tone is normal, the examiner should feel the patient's fingers vibrating together upon more rigorous shaking. Have the patient extend and supinate both arms (Fig. 3.8), then observe for pronator drift while his eyes are closed.

Pronation during this maneuver suggests upper motor neuron type weakness. Depression or instability may indicate ipsilateral cerebellar disease. Choreiform and dystonic abnormal movements may also manifest themselves during this test, as may postural tremors.

The examiner may move from this maneuver to a formal assessment of cerebellar function on finger-to-nose testing. Remember that it is more difficult

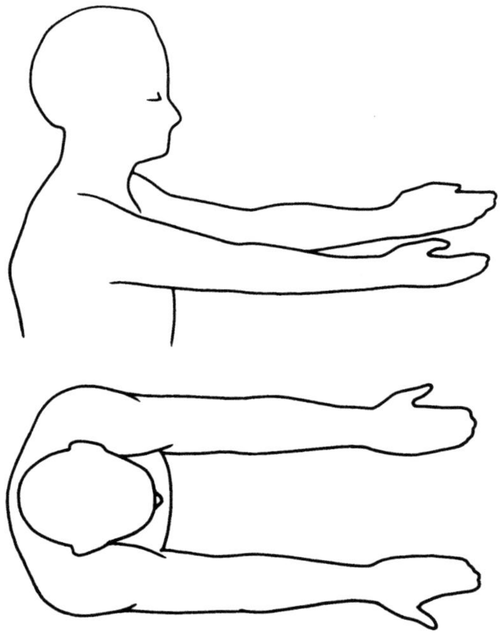

**Figure 3.8.** Test for pronator drift.

to perform this movement slowly than quickly. Grip strength in either hand should be checked at this point. For those who are unable to resist the urge to perform individual muscle strength testing, the time to do so has arrived at this point.

## Lower Extremities

We prefer to assess leg strength, tone, and coordination in the sitting position, examiner facing patient. Tone in the lower extremities is not well assessed in this position (see "Reflexes") except for ankle clonus, which may be elicited by sharply dorsiflexing the patient's foot. The strength of more proximal hip girdle musculature may be screened by assessing flexion, abduction, and abduction of the upper leg against resistance (Fig. 3.9).

The patient's ability to slide the heel of one leg down the shin of the other is tested next. The correct performance of this test draws on complex motor and cerebellar systems. Again, beware of the patient who compensates for a subtle deficit by performing the test quickly.

## Abnormal Movements

Throughout the motor examination, the psychiatrist is on the alert for evidence of movement disorders. Scales exist for quantifying various abnormal movements, but few are as useful as a clear description. The following definitions of abnormal movements are provided as a suggested outline to organize such descriptions.

*Tremor.* Oscillating, rapid movement, usually more distal than proximal. Describe amplitude (''course'' or ''fine''), and estimate rate. Describe whether it is exacerbated or improved by rest, posture, or action.

*Chorea.* Irregular movements, erratic in amplitude and speed, but usually quick and darting. These movements are usually more distal than proximal—the ''dance.'' Describe which limbs are affected and how severely.

*Dystonia.* A more proximal, sometimes tonic abnormal movement, commonly producing what looks like abnormal posture. Torticollis is one of the dystonias. Again, describe which muscle groups are involved and how severely.

*Athetosis.* A more distal, slow and writhing abnormal movement, which may produce bizarre posturing of distal extremities. Athetosis is commonly intermingled with chorea, in which case the term ''choreoathetoid'' may be applied.

*Ballism.* A proximal, high-amplitude, rapid movement of extremities which appears ''flinging'' in nature. This particular movement is rare among psychiatric patients but may occasionally be seen as part of tardive dyskinesia.

*Myoclonus.* Lightninglike focal contraction of muscle groups of sufficient strength to produce movement across a joint. These ''jerks'' may involve seg-

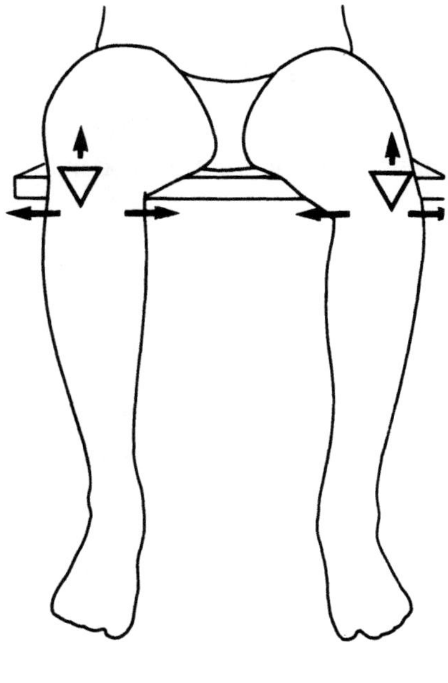

**Figure 3.9.** Directions of resistance in hip girdle strength.

mental muscles of the trunk ("spinal myoclonus") or more distal muscle groups. Some of the myoclonic syndromes are forms of epilepsy, and some are related to metabolic, spinal cord, or brainstem pathology.

## REFLEXES

The muscle stretch reflexes are based on monosynaptic circuits but influenced by a variety of peripheral and more central systems. Observations on these reflexes tend to be more objective and a bit less experience-dependent than observations in other areas of the neurologic examination, but considerable variation still exists as a function of age, sex, and emotional state. With reluctance, we have concluded over the years that left/right asymmetries of reflex response may exist on a conversion basis. We suggest the following initial examination.

### Upper Extremities

The muscle stretch reflexes in the upper extremity may be well examined at the conclusion of the upper-extremity motor examination, while patient and examiner are seated and facing each other. Three reflexes are examined: brachioradialis (C5, 6), biceps (C5, 6), and triceps (C6, 7, 8) as in Fig. 3.10. If the examiner holds the patient's relaxed forearms by the thumbs, more accurate left/right comparisons may be made. The reflexes should be recorded on a stick figure in the chart according to the outline in Fig. 3.11.

### Lower Extremities

Lower-extremity reflexes are best graded during the portion of the examination (general medical, abdominal) when the patient is lying supine on the

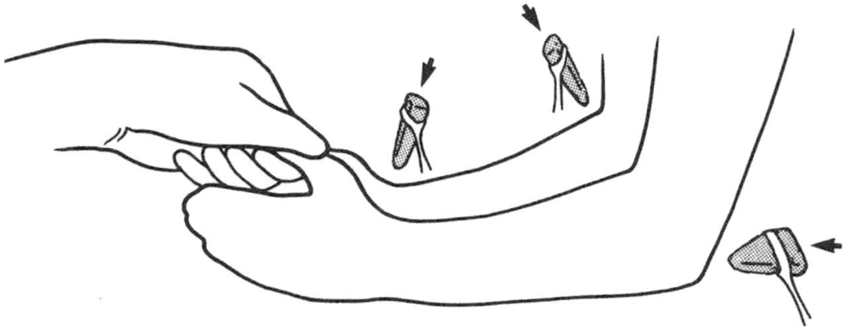

**Figure 3.10.** Muscle stretch reflexes in arms.

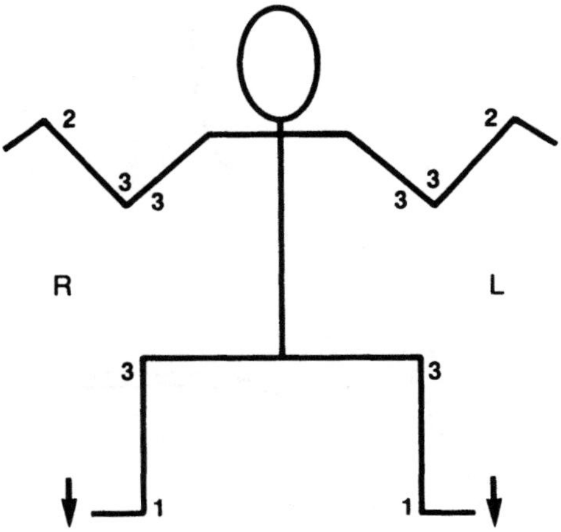


**Figure 3.11.** Format for recording muscle stretch reflexes. O, No response; 1, present but reduced; 2, normal; 3, brisk, possibly pathological; 4, clonus present, pathological.

examination table. Muscle tone in the lower extremities may also be examined to advantage in this position. The examiner assists the patient in relaxing as much as possible, and then gently flexes and extends each leg at the knee. If tone is normal, the heel will track along the surface of the examination table. If tone is increased, the heel may extend from the surface of the table. The knee jerk reflexes (L2, 3, 4) are best examined with the legs symmetrically flexed at approximately 60° (as opposed to 90° in the sitting position) (Fig. 3.12). Very accurate side/side comparisons may be made.

The ankle jerks (S1) may be tested in the same position after rotating the leg, externally on the hip, so that it lies flat upon the table, and dorsiflexing the foot to apply some tension to the Achilles' tendon.

## Babinski Sign

Although not a muscle stretch reflex, plantar stimulation to the foot is customarily applied after the lower-extremity reflexes are graded (Fig. 3.13).

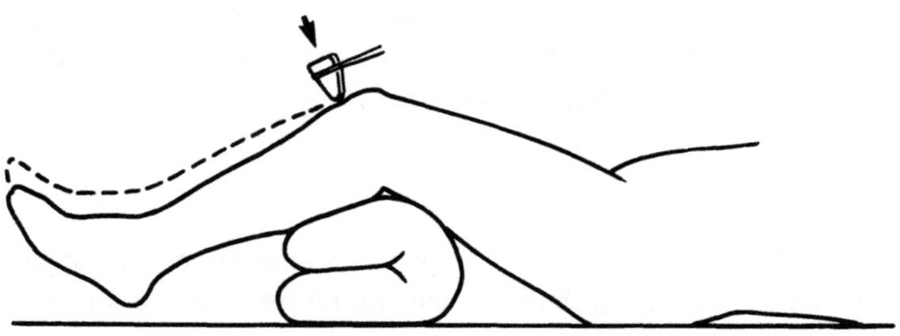

**Figure 3.12.** Position for examining knee jerk reflexes.

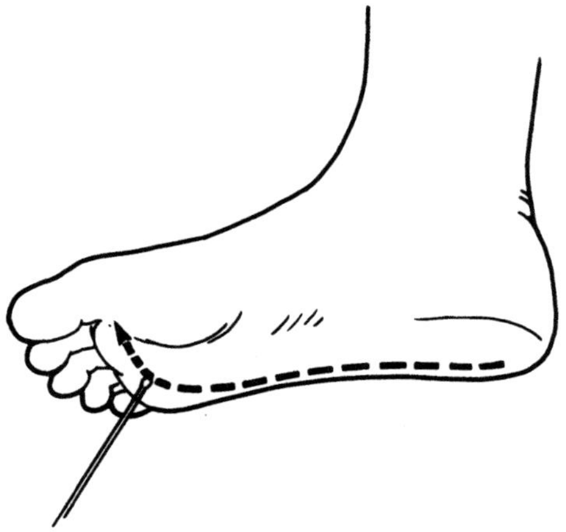

**Figure 3.13.** Method for eliciting Babinski sign.

A blunted point should be used. Remember that, although the complete Babinski response includes dorsiflexion of the great toe, fanning of the other toes, and flexion withdrawal of the leg, only dorsiflexion of the great toe may be present. When judgment is difficult, observe the great toe carefully for its *first* motion after the first or second plantar stimulus.

## RELEASE SIGNS

It is uncertain whether the so-called disinhibitory signs of "frontal release" signs are of localizing or diagnostic value. There are a number of clinical publications concerning their association with neurologic diseases that involve both hemispheres diffusely (Paulson and Gottlieb, 1968; Joynt *et al.*, 1962; Granacher, 1981; Fink *et al.*, 1952; Jenkyn *et al.*, 1977), but an unacceptable number of false-positive and negative results may be associated with any single sign. In addition, the impact of normal aging on the reappearance of these signs (most of them were present at one time during infantile development) has not been studied sufficiently. On the other hand, it is our clinical impression that the appearance of two or more of these signs is suggestive for the diagnosis of diffuse cerebral disease. We recommend the following four tests in our screening neurologic examination.

### Snout Response

A tongue blade is placed across the patient's relaxed lips and tapped gently with the reflex hammer (Fig. 3.14). A pursing response of the lips is the positive sign.

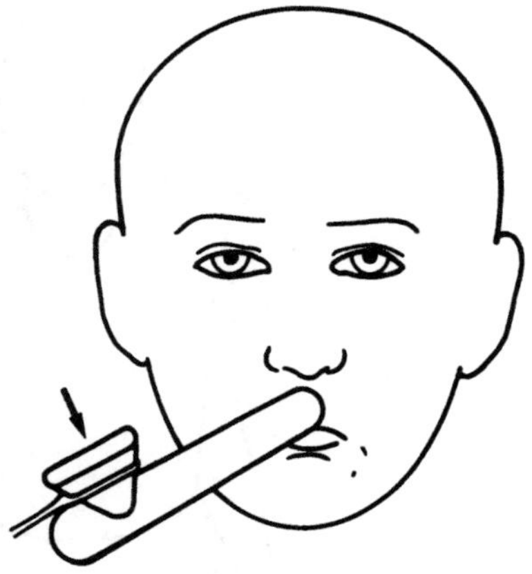

**Figure 3.14.** Elicitation of snout response.

## Grasp Response

The examiner grasps the patient's corresponding hand, palm against palm, as in shaking hands. He then gently disengages his hand by sliding it out of the patient's grasp. The positive response consists in a continuing, sometimes quite forceful grasp by the patient. The response is most reliably elicited while the patient's attention is distracted. Occasionally, a continuing grasp response may be confused with willful handshaking, but in our experience such confusion usually belongs to the examiner.

## Nuchocephalic Response

The patient is assisted to relax in a seated position facing the examiner (Fig. 3.15). The examiner firmly grasps both shoulders and asks the patient to close his eyes. The patient's shoulders are then quickly rotated 20° in either direction. The normal response is for the head and neck to "follow" the shoulders around in a supple motion after a brief delay. When the abnormal response is present, the patient's head and neck remain in the forward-facing position, or turn en bloc with the shoulders.

## Paratonia

In normal muscle tone, there is some minimal resistance felt by the examiner through range of motion testing, which is roughly equal throughout the arc of the motion. With increased tone from extrapyramidal syndromes (i.e., parkinsonism), the resistance is increased, almost leaden, throughout the move-

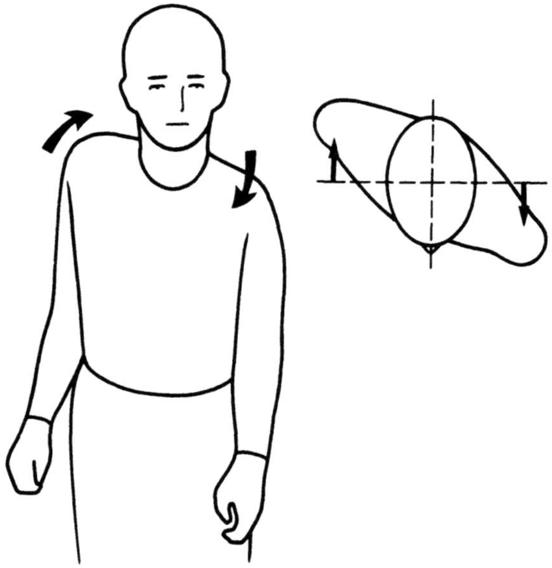

**Figure 3.15.** Elicitation of nuchocephalic response.

ment arc. In spasticity, there is velocity-dependent hypertonus, which appears as a "catch" when the passive range of motion is suddenly accelerated. The best description of paratonia is that "it is like none of these." In paratonia, there is a disconcerting mix of too much and too little. The patient may briefly seem to be helping the examiner (*mitgehen*) and in the next moment working against him (*gegenhalten*). The only distinction of difficulty is when the paratonia is severe, when it can be mistaken for "lead pipe" hypertonus. As in so many other areas of examination, patient and repeated observations will reveal periods of *mitgehen* along with the *gegenhalten*. Some advanced Alzheimer's patients do have extrapyramidal tone abnormalities, but a number of them receive L-dopa as a treatment for the paratonia. The clinician soon learns that L-dopa does not significantly improve Alzheimer's disease.

## SENSORY EXAMINATION

The sensory examination is placed last in this clinical outline, since it is not often useful in psychiatric patients. For that matter, it is the least reliable portion of the neurologic examination for *any* patient population. We suggest that it be performed quickly and with élan, so that no ponderousness becomes attached to the results, either by patient or physician. One test from each of the following modalities should be examined, with the most careful attention directed to left/right and distal/proximal differences in stimulus perception.

## Pin Sensation

Selected dermatomes should be sampled in arm, leg, and face, emphasizing perceived differences between left and right. If the patient reports such a difference, ask which side is normal? On the first examination, attempt only rough caudal/cephalad and left/right outlines of the deficit area.

## Light Touch

The receptors for light touch and the central transmission may be a bit different from those for pain or pin sensation. A white cotton Q-tip is a good instrument to use.

## Vibration

Use a 128-cps tuning fork, applied to the soft-tissue portion of one digit from each extremity. Keep the fork off bony surfaces, since the vibration can be transmitted up the ossicular chain to be perceived at a more proximal level. A simple way to perform the test is to apply the vibrating fork and ask the patient to acknowledge the sensation. As the vibration decays, ask the patient to indicate the point of its subjective disappearance. The examiner compares this with his own perception and experience.

## Proprioception

This is tested by flexing or extending the distal interphalangeal joint of a finger or toe. Ask the patient to keep his eyes closed and identify the direction of movement either up or down.

## Cortical Sensation

It is somewhat artificial to associate a specific clinical test with a specific level of the neuraxis, but there is a series of more complex sensory tests that require intact cerebral hemispheric function for their correct interpretation. These include graphesthesia, double simultaneous stimulation, two-point discrimination, and stereognosis. These need not be performed routinely. The clinician may select one of them to use when hemispheric or parietal lobe dysfunction is suspected and to develop familiarity with this test. Graphesthesia testing is illustrated as one example:

*Physician:* "I am going to write some numbers on the tips of your fingers, which I want you to judge with your eyes closed. The numbers will be facing you, as if on a blackboard."

Three successive numbers are applied to the left hand, followed by three to the right. The number of correct responses from the patient is recorded. The number "5" may be the most difficult and should be among the numbers applied to both hands. Beware of a pattern of error that improves when the second hand is tested. This may indicate test-related learning or opposed-to-true unilateral hemispheric dysfunction.

## REFERENCES


Adams, R. D., and Victor, M. *Principles of Neurology,* 3d ed. New York: McGraw-Hill, 1985.

Anderson, W. H. The physical examination in office practice. *Am. J. Psychiatry,* 1980, **137,** 1188–1192.

Baker, A. B., and Joynt, R. J. (eds.). *Clinical Neurology,* revised edition. Philadelphia: Harper and Row, 1986.

Beresford, T. P., Blow F. C., Nichols, L. O., and Langston, J. W. Focal signs and brain CT scans in psychiatric patients. *N. Engl. J. Med.,* 1985, **313,** 388 (letter).

Cummings, J. L. *Clinical Neuropsychiatry.* Orlando, FL: Grune and Stratton, 1985.

DeJong, R. N. *The Neurologic Examination,* 4th ed. Hagerstown, MD: Harper and Row, 1979.

Denes, G., Semenza, C., Stoppa, E., and Lis, A. Unilateral spatial neglect and recovery from hemiplegia: A follow-up study. *Brain,* 1982, **105,** 543–552.

Fink, M., Green, M., and Bender, M. B. The face–hand test as a diagnostic sign of organic mental syndrome. *Neurology,* 1952, **2,** 46–58.

Geschwind, N. Aphasia. *N. Engl. J. Med.,* 1971, **284,** 654–656.

Granacher, R. P. The neurologic examination in geriatric psychiatry. *Psychosomatics,* 1981, **22,** 485–499.

Jenkyn, L. R., Walsh D. B., Culver, C. M., and Reeves, A. G. Clinical signs in diffuse cerebral dysfunction. *J. Neurol. Neurosurg. Psychiatry,* 1977, **40,** 956–966.

Joynt, R. J., Benton, A. L. and Fogel, M. L. Behavioral and pathological correlates of motor impersistence. *Neurology,* 1962, **12,** 876–881.

Larson, E. B., Mack, L. A., Watts, B., and Cromwell, L. D. Computed tomography in patients with psychiatric illnesses: Advantage of a "rule-in" approach. *Ann. Intern. Med.,* 1981, **95,** 360–364.

Lezak, M. D. *Neuropsychological Assessment,* 2d ed. New York: Oxford University Press, 1983.

Luria, A. R. *Higher Cortical Functions in Man,* 2d ed. New York: Basic Books, 1966.

Lynch G., McGaugh, J. L., and Weinberger, N. M. (eds.). *Neurobiology of Learning and Memory.* New York: Guilford Press, 1984.

Mancall, E. L. *Alpers and Mancall's Essentials of the Neurologic Examination,* 2d ed. Philadelphia: F. A. Davis, 1981.

Medical Research Council. *Aids to the Investigation of Peripheral Nerve Injuries.* London: Her Majesty's Stationery Office, 1943.

Mesulam, M.-M. A cortical network for directed attention and unilateral neglect. *Ann. Neurol.,* 1981, **10,** 309–325.

Mesulam, M.-M. *Principles of Behavioral Neurology.* Philadelphia: F. A. Davis, 1985.

Miller, N. R. (ed.). *Walsh and Hoyt's Clinical Neuro-Ophthalmology,* ed. IV, Vol. I. Baltimore: Williams and Wilkins, 1982.

Mukherjee, S., Shukla, J., and Rosen, A. Neurological abnormalities in patients with bipolar disorder. *Biol. Psychiatry,* 1984, **19,** 337–345.

Papez, J. W. A proposed mechanism of emotion. *Arch. Neurol. Psychol.,* 1937, **38,** 725–743.

Paulson, G., and Gottlieb, G. Development reflexes: The reappearance of fetal and neonatal reflexes in aged patients. *Brain,* 1968, **91,** 37–52.

Plum, F., and Posner, J. B. *The Diagnosis of Stupor and Coma,* 3d ed. Philadelphia: F. A. Davis, 1980.

Reiser, D. E., and Schroder, A. K. *Patient Interviewing: The Human Dimension.* Baltimore: Williams and Wilkins, 1980.

Rowland, L. P. (ed.). *Merritt's Textbook of Neurology,* 7th Ed. Philadelphia: Lea and Febiger, 1984.

Schiffer, R. B., Herndon, R. M., and Rudick, R. A. Treatment of pathologic laughing and weeping with amitriptyline. *N. Engl. J. Med.,* 1985, **312,** 1480–1482.

Strub, R. L., and Black, F. W. *The Mental Status Examination in Neurology,* 2d ed. Philadelphia: F. A. Davis, 1985.

Summers, W. K., Munoz, R. A., Read, M. R., and Marsh, G. M. The psychiatric physical examination. II. Findings in 72 unselected psychiatric patients. *J. Clin. Psychiatry,* 1981, **42,** 99–102.

Tucker, G. J., Campion, E. W., and Silberfarb, P. M. Sensorimotor functions and cognitive disturbance in psychiatric patients. *Am. J. Psychiatry,* 1975, **132,** 17–21.

Van Allen, M. W., and Rodnitzky, R. L. *Pictorial Manual of Neurologic Tests,* 2d ed. Chicago: Year Book, 1981.

Wells, C. E., and Duncan G. W. *Neurology for Psychiatrists.* Philadelphia: F. A. Davis, 1980.

Wiederholt, W. C. (ed.). *Neurology for Non-Neurologists.* New York: Academic Press, 1982.

Woods, B. T., Kinney, D. K., and Yurgelun-Todd, D. Neurologic abnormalities in schizophrenic patients and their families. I. Comparison of schizophrenic, bipolar, and substance abuse patients and normal controls. *Arch. Gen. Psychiatry,* 1986, **43,** 657–663.

# 4

# General Physical Examination

## THE INTERVIEW IN PREPARATION FOR THE PHYSICAL EXAMINATION

It is impossible to discuss the physical examination without a consideration of the interview that precedes it. The interview broadly generates data concerning the individual patient which permits the examiner to formulate hypotheses to be tested through the physical examination, laboratory testing, and further investigations.

The interview should be conducted with patient and examiner seated at the same level and with the patient adequately clothed and comfortable. The pace should be slow, especially at the beginning of the interview and with the elderly patient. A period of open-ended questioning is extremely valuable in assessing mental status and in facilitating patient participation.

### Present Illness

The presenting clinical problem or illness should always be assumed to have a dimension that will be manifest in somatic symptoms. The degree to which the patient pays attention to his or her bodily functioning during psychiatric illness will influence responses when the interviewer asks open-ended questions such as "Tell me how you've been feeling." For this reason, more focused questions may be necessary early in the interview, such as "Have you felt any physical problems or symptoms during the time you've been sick or recently?" "Have you felt any bodily discomfort since this problem began?" Positive answers to such questions must be followed by more inquiry to elicit the characteristics of somatic symptoms, since these characteristics will be the key to the pathophysiology underlying the symptom.

The patient's exact description of the symptom may also supply evidence for various somatization processes such as conversion reactions, hypochondriasis, or somatic delusions. Recording of the patient's verbal descriptors is valuable here. Manic patients may deny or minimize somatic symptoms or medical history. The interviewer may need to repeat some specific questions at different points in the interview and seek independent sources of information from relatives or medical records. Conversely, the depressed patient may focus on somatic symptoms or function. This may result in a large number of symptoms elaborately described or preoccupation with a single symptom. It is also true that biologically induced changes in somatic function in depression are responsible for anorexia, constipation, sleep disturbances, and weight loss.

After eliciting the history of current somatic symptoms, the interviewer should establish whether there has been a disruption of food or fluid intake, sleep, and physical activity. Food and fluid intake may be disrupted by anorexia, disturbances of consciousness, substitution by alcohol or drugs, excitement, or apathy. Weight loss, vitamin deficiencies, weakness, dehydration, orthostatic hypotension, and electrolyte disturbance may be present depending on the duration of the disruption. As in other areas of inquiry, it may be necessary to have the reports of family or significant others who have observed the patient in order to elicit this information. Sleep and physical activity levels during the present illness will be affected by the patient's mood, presence of agitation, and excitement or apathy but also by the presence of limiting physical factors such as pain, injuries to extremities, muscular rigidity, or weakness. Rarely, extreme muscular exertion occurs during psychotic states and may lead to exhaustion, muscle tenderness, and breakdown with myoglobinuria and extreme elevations of plasma creatine phosphokinase (CPK) activity (Weiner, 1985).

Inquiry concerning the use of medications is important in order to learn about drug-induced symptoms or relief of symptoms and to guide the search for drug-induced physical or mental status findings. This inquiry should include all drugs, including tobacco, psychotropic medications, "medical" prescriptions for concurrent medical problems and over-the-counter preparations. Dosages and frequency of use are important clues to drug or prescription abuse, doctor shopping, and dependence on chemicals. Gathering data about medication usage also helps in assessing the patient's interpretation and understanding of his or her illness.

Answers to questions concerning the pattern of professional contacts and efforts at treatment of the presenting illness will give clues about the extent to which physical factors have been evaluated or treated in the illness. Often the first or sole professional contact has been with a nonmedical therapist. The patient may have been referred by his primary care physician. If this is the case, it is still necessary to carefully evaluate somatic factors, since the perspective of the psychiatric examiner will be quite different and will influence the meaning assigned to somatic symptoms and process.

Special attention must be paid to the history of alcohol and illicit drug use during the present illness and to the pattern of alcohol and drug use prior to illness. Denial and minimization are frequent forms of resistance here, and the interviewer will need to be aware of this factor. A second interview with a significant other is always a good step in this area of inquiry.

## Past History

After eliciting data concerning the present illness a review of the past health and illness history will help to focus hypotheses for the examiner to pursue in the physical examination. A question concerning the patient's perception of his or her overall health must be followed by specific inquiries regarding prior hospitalizations, operations, injuries, childbirth and gynecologic treatment, primary health care provider contacts, and known disabilities or chronic illnesses (e.g., diabetes, hypertension, anemia, arthritis, epilepsy). All of these illnesses have potential physical findings. Apart from the specific facts concerning past illness episodes, this area of inquiry should give the examiner a sense of the patient's level of knowledge and concern about his or her health and the status of relationships with physicians or health care providers and the level of coordination between these health care providers. Frequently, the examiner will feel the need to document further the facts obtained in this portion of the history by contacting other care providers (with the patient's permission).

## Family History

Eliciting the history of health and illness in the patient's family is essential to opening up hypotheses concerning the nature of the patient's own illnesses past, present, and future. A general question such as "Are there any diseases or conditions that run in your family?" needs to be followed by mention of specific medical and psychiatric disorders such as coronary artery disease, epilepsy, hypertension, diabetes, alcoholism, depressive illness, schizophrenia, and premature death from any cause. There are by-products of this area of inquiry in the form of data concerning the patient's relationships within the family and the patient's degree of concern over his or her own health vis-à-vis the known familial disorders. For example, the grief process following death of a close relative may have important implications for the patient's present state of health; fear of developing diabetes or heart disease, like their close relative, may contribute to stress.

The examiner should be able to draw or diagram the family for three generations concerning major diseases, cause, and age at death. Such a diagram can be a starting point for further exploration of family factors in the psychiatric illness.

## Personal and Social History

By using a developmental framework to review the occurrence of specific illnesses, the examiner can develop facts to be pursued during a physical examination. For example, childhood illnesses such as rheumatic fever, renal disease, and attention deficit disorder may leave physical and psychological residua. Physical trauma in adolescence or early adulthood may leave physical disfiguration, functional disabilities, and body image distortions or low self-esteem. Physical growth and development including puberty and menarche are examples of somatic processes that have physical and emotional implications. Geographical moves may produce exposure to infectious diseases or other environmental health hazards. Marriage, procreation, and occupation have physical and emotional health implications. This area of inquiry serves not only as an orientation for the physical examination but also for hypotheses about psychological adaptation. In this era of rising prevalence rates for human immune deficiency virus infections, the patient's sexual behavior should be discussed.

## Review of Systems

This inquiry is used to complete the survey of symptoms or problems related to present and past health. It serves to stimulate recall in patients who tend to minimize or deny symptoms. It may also bring out hypochondriacal symptom patterns. A useful sequence of symptom inquiry is by a combination of region and systems, such as head, eyes, ears, nose, throat, neck, respiratory, cardiovascular, gastrointestinal (including nutrition), genitourinary (including sexual function), musculoskeletal, neurologic, and skin.

The total duration of the interview preceding the physical examination will vary depending on the circumstances and goals of the examination. If the examiner has 1 hr to devote to the interview and physical examination, we suggest 45 min for interviewing and 15 min for the physical examination. Of course, 1 hr is not adequate to perform a comprehensive assessment of the psychiatric patient, and we assume that additional interviews will be performed, before or after the physical examination.

# PHYSICAL EXAMINATION

When the interview has been completed, the examiner should inform the patient that the next procedure is a physical examination and request the patient to undress and put on the gown provided. In the hospital inpatient service, a floor nurse may have already supervised the patient's dressing for the examination. It is important to provide privacy for the patient to undress; a curtain partition in the office or examining room serves this purpose. In some instances it will be appropriate to have a nurse assist during the examination. This is particularly important if the patient is seductive, frightened, intoxicated, psychotic, or likely to misinterpret the nature of the examination. In all instances a female nurse should assist during the female pelvic examination.

Table 4.1 and Fig. 4.1 illustrate a sequence of examiner–patient positions

**Table 4.1**
Summary of the Examiner's and Patient's Positions during Physical Examination of the Ambulatory Patient[a]

| Region | Examiner's position | Patient's position |
|---|---|---|
| 1. General inspection and vital signs | Standing before the patient and moving as needed | Sitting, or lying on the bed or examining table |
| 2. Head | Standing, facing the patient | Sitting on the side of the bed or examining table |
| 3. Neck | Standing, facing the patient, then moving behind him | Sitting on the side of the bed or examining table |
| 4. Back; posterior thorax and lungs | Standing behind the patient | Sitting on the side of the bed or examining table |
| 5. Anterior thorax and lungs | Standing, facing the patient | Sitting on the side of the bed or examining table |
| 6. Breasts and axillary regions | Initially facing the patient, then examining from the patient's right side | Sitting, facing the examiner, then lying supine |
| 7. Heart | Standing at the patient's right | In three positions: sitting, lying on his back, and lying on his left side |
| 8. Abdomen | Standing at the patient's right | Lying on his back |
| 9. Extremities | Standing, facing the patient, and moving to the patient's right | Lying flat, then sitting on the side of the bed, and finally standing |
| 10. Male external genitalia | Standing before the patient and slightly to his right | Standing, facing the examiner |
| 11. Female genital tract | Sitting on a stool facing the perineum, and standing for part of the examination | Lying on her back on an examining table with both knees flexed and feet in stirrups |
| 12. Rectum | Standing, facing the buttocks | Bending at the hips over the bed or examining table. The female retains the same position used in the examination of the genital tract |

[a]From Morgan and Engel (1969), with permission.

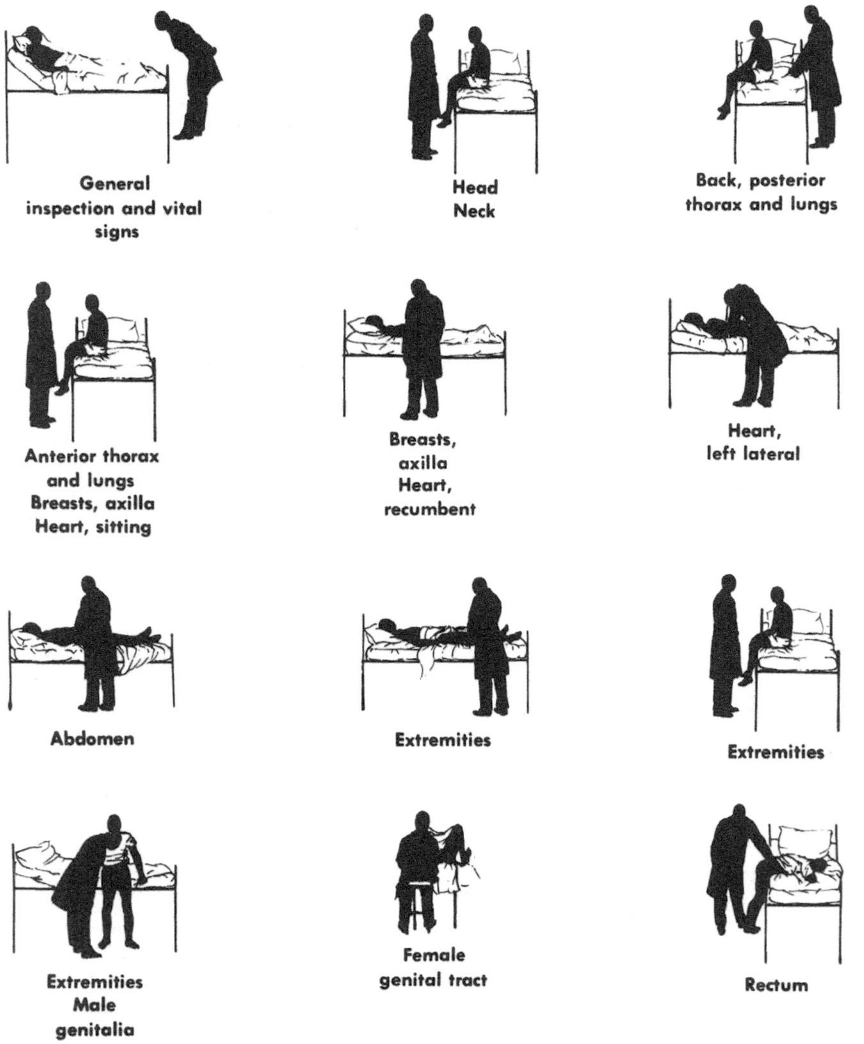


**Figure 4.1.** The ambulatory patient. (From Morgan and Engel, 1969, with permission.)

that facilitate a complete physical examination for the ambulatory patient. The following description of a physical examination will be in this sequence. Some systems, such as skin and lymph nodes, are examined regionally throughout the entire sequence. Because of the special relevance of the neurological examination to evaluation of the psychiatric patient, we have described it separately in Chapter 3. The neurological system can also be examined regionally throughout the complete physical examination.

The reader is referred to several texts for details of techniques of examination (Morgan and Engel, 1969; Burnside and McGlynn, 1987; DeGowin, 1987; Delp and Manning, 1981; Bates, 1987). The following is a statement of the general physical examination we use for most psychiatric inpatients and outpatients. In some instances, more specialized and detailed examination using specialists will be indicated following the general examination.

## Position 1

The examination should begin with the patient seated on an examining table or bed and the examiner facing the patient and observing for posture, movements, facial expression and symmetry, and degree of tension or relaxation.

### Vital Signs

The oral temperature should be taken if it is not already recorded. Blood pressure should be taken in both arms and should be repeated with the patient standing if there is concern about present or future orthostatic hypotension. The heart rate and respiratory rate can be counted after the blood pressure is recorded.

### HEENT

The skull is palpated and the scalp is inspected, particularly at the margins for signs of seborrhea.

The eyes are inspected for symmetry and presence of stare or lid lag. Test for range of extraocular movements, pupil size, symmetry, and reaction. Examine fundus with ophthalmoscope, and observe optic discs, arteries, veins, and retinae.

Inspect the ears including pinnae and external auditory canals. Using the otoscope, examine the tympanic membranes.

Test for nasal obstruction by having the patient sniff. Examine the interior of nasal passages using a speculum and light. Examine the nasal septum.

Inspect the mouth for missing teeth, caries, or gingival disorders. Inspect oral mucosa, pharynx, uvula, tonsillar area, and tongue.

Inspect the neck for symmetry and gross nodules. Have the patient swallow during inspection to observe for thyroid enlargement or masses.

Palpate for lymph nodes, tracheal position, and thyroid size, shape, and consistency. Confirmation of thyroid palpation should be done with the examiner standing behind the patient.

Test range of neck motion during flexion, extension, and lateral flexion.

Palpate and auscultate carotid arteries singly.

## Position 2

The examiner then moves to stand behind the patient and exposes the posterior thorax. Inspect chest and spine for asymmetry or deformity. Palpate for tactile fremitus while the patient vocalizes test words. Perform percussion of the thorax to establish resonance level and position of diaphragms. Auscultate for breath sounds, rales, and rhonchi before and after coughing.

## Position 3

Facing the patient, the examiner then exposes anterior thorax, using appropriate cover for breasts of female patient until examination of that region.

Inspect anterior thorax, heart, breasts, and upper extremities.

Inspect, percuss, and auscultate the anterior thorax to include the lateral thorax and axillary regions. Inspect the precordium for impulses. Palpate for thrills and point of maximal impulse. Auscultate heart sounds, murmurs, and gallops at the apex and base of heart.

Inspect both breasts with arms elevated. Look for asymmetry, skin changes, nipple deformity.

Inspect the upper extremities for scars, needle track sites, tattoos. Inspect hands. Palpate axillary and epitrochlear areas. Test the motion of all upper extremity joints.

## Position 4

The patient lies down, and the examiner now stands at patient's right side.

### Completion of Cardiac and Breast Examinations

The precordium is again palpated for the point of maximal impact. Auscultation of heart sounds and murmurs is repeated with patient tilting to left lateral decubitus position.

The breast examination is facilitated by having the patient place her hand under her head and placing a small pillow or folded sheet under the scapula on the side being examined. Both maneuvers elevate the chest wall and allow more even distribution of breast tissue over the thorax. Palpate the entire breast for masses and nipple discharge.

### Abdomen

Inspect the entire undraped abdomen for symmetry and contour. Palpate gently, then deeply in all four quadrants, searching for abnormal masses, contours, and tenderness.

Palpate for hepatic margin, splenic margin, and aortic impulse. Percuss upper and lower margins of the liver.

Auscultate for bruits, especially in lower quadrants. Auscultate for bowel sounds.

The inguinal region should be palpated for lymph nodes and femoral artery pulsations.

### Lower Extremities

Inspect both legs including the feet. Test movements at all lower extremity joints. Palpate knee and ankle joints. Palpate for pedal edema. Palpate for pedal pulses and calf tenderness.

## Position 5

Patient resumes a sitting position with the examiner facing the patient. Ask the patient to stand, offering necessary assistance.

Inspect lower extremities, spine, male genitalia, and the male rectal area.

Inspect for varicosities, feet pronation, and stance.

Inspect the spine for contour. Test for range of motion and presence of pain with movement.

Inspect and palpate the penis, testes, and scrotum; search for inguinal herniae.

## Position 6

With male patient bending at hip level to rest upper body on examining table or bed and examiner facing buttocks, inspect the buttocks including cleft and anus. Insert lubricated gloved finger into rectum for palpation of entire circumference of rectum and prostate gland. Obtain stool sample on gloved finger to test for occult blood.

## Position 7

With female patient recumbent on examining table with legs flexed and feet in stirrups, inspect perineal region and external genitalia. Palpate inguinal region for nodes if not done during abdominal examination. Using unlubricated speculum, inspect the vagina and cervix. Obtain cytological specimens from the cervix and vagina. Withdraw speculum; insert lubricated fingers into vagina for bimanual examination, palpating uterus and adnexal regions. Perform rectovaginal confirmatory examination, and obtain gloved-finger stool sample for occult blood testing.

## POSTEXAMINATION INTERVIEW

Following the physical examination, when the patient has assumed a comfortable sitting position and has dressed, there should be a brief interview dealing with the patient's questions about the examination results and including a statement to the patient about how positive physical findings or medical issues will be considered in the development of an evaluation and treatment plan. The examiner can indicate to the patient that laboratory test results will be discussed when they are available. The examiner can also emphasize that subsequent interviews or meetings will deal in more depth with the details of the behavorial and emotional aspects of the patient's presenting problem. Such a statement will return the focus of the relationship to the most relevant issues.

If the patient is unable to comprehend the nature or purpose of the examination because of psychosis, delirium, or dementia, the interview after the examination should be more reassuring and less factual, and further information processing may have to be postponed or omitted.

## PATIENT–EXAMINER RELATIONSHIP

In situations where the examiner has serious concerns about transference and countertransference reactions to the physical examination, arrangements should be made for a different person to perform the physical examination. This would still allow the primary clinician to obtain the medical history through the interview process as described and to integrate the results of the physical examination into the diagnostic and treatment plan. In the authors' experience the initial comprehensive assessment including medical history and physical examination does not create serious transference–countertransference problems in most psychiatric patients. In long-term therapy or intensive psychotherapy, it may be that distortion of the psychotheraputic relationship is produced by a physical examination. The data bearing on this issue have been discussed in Chapter 1, and it remains a matter of clinical judgment. As stated there, we suspect that much more general medical or neurologic care may be carried out within the context of the psychotherapeutic relationship than is customarily conducted at the present time.

## REFERENCES

Bates, B. *A Guide to Physical Examination and History Taking,* 5th ed. Philadelphia: Lippincott, 1987.

Burnside, J. W., and McGlynn, T. J. *Physical Diagnosis,* 17th ed. Baltimore: Williams & Wilkins, 1987.

DeGowin, R. L. *DeGowin and DeGowin's Bedside Diagnostic Examination*, 5th ed. New York: Macmillan, 1987.

Delp, M. H., and Manning, R. T. *Major's Physical Diagnosis*. Philadelphia: W. B. Saunders, 1981.

Morgan, W. L., and Engel, G. L. *The Clinical Approach to the Patient*. Philadelphia: W. B. Saunders, 1969.

Weiner, H. Schizophrenia, etiology. In Kaplan, H. I., and Sadock, B. J. (eds.): *Comprehensive Textbook of Psychiatry*, Vol. IV. Baltimore: Williams & Wilkins, 1985.

# 5

# Depressive Syndrome

### DSM-III-R Diagnoses

*Major Depressive Syndrome.* An illness episode characterized by either depressed mood, or loss of interest or pleasure. The illness episode should be further characterized by at least five psychobiologic signs of depression, such as weight change, sleep disturbance, psychomotor changes, anergy, feelings of worthlessness, impaired concentration, or recurrent thoughts of death.

*Dysthymia.* An illness characterized by chronically depressed mood for at least two years.

*Adjustment Disorder with Depressed Mood.* A reaction to an identifiable psychosocial stressor which is characterized by depressed mood, tearfulness, or hopelessness.

### ICD-9 Diagnoses

*Manic Depressive Psychosis, Depressed Type.* An affective psychosis in which there is a widespread depressed mood of gloom and wretchedness with some degree of anxiety. There is often reduced activity but there may be restlessness and agitation. There is a marked tendency to recurrence; in a few cases this may be at regular intervals.

*Neurotic Depression.* A neurotic disorder characterized by disproportionate depression which has usually recognizably ensued on a distressing experience; it does not include among its features delusions or hallucinations, and there is often preoccupation with the psychic trauma which preceded the illness, e.g., loss of a cherished person or possession. Anxiety is also frequently present and mixed states of anxiety and depression should be included here.

*Neurasthenia.* A neurotic disorder characterized by fatigue, irritability, headache, depression, insomnia, difficulty in concentration, and lack of capacity for enjoyment (anhedonia). It may follow or accompany an infection or exhaustion, or arise from continued emotional stress.

We are reminded at the beginning of this, our longest chapter, that the brain has a peculiar propensity toward depressive feelings. When Denis Williams interviewed 100 epileptic patients who had experienced ictal emotions, he found that the vast majority reported pessimistic, dysphoric, or apprehensive feelings (Williams, 1956). And when Gloor *et al.* reported the results of his stimulation experiments in the brains of wakeful humans, they stated that pleasurable sensations were but rarely evoked (Gloor *et al.*, 1982). A similar circumstance seems to hold for cats and monkeys (Anand and Dua, 1955). Cheerful, pleasurable, and upbeat emotions were sometimes elicited from septal regions in these studies, but such feelings seem distinctly less common and more difficult to "find" with the searching electrode than the darker emotions. One might speculate that the central nervous system (CNS) is physiologically predisposed to respond nonspecifically to a variety of insults with sadness.

There are two other complicating factors that make clinical diagnosis particularly difficult with regard to depressive affective syndromes. One is that a wide array of medical and neurologic diseases commonly generate vague somatic symptoms early in their course that are "depressionlike." In particular, sensations of vague discomfort, fatigue, and lassitude occur early in extra-CNS metabolic and musculoskeletal disorders. Warnes (1982) has provided a list of such disorders (Table 5.1).

**Table 5.1**
Medical Diseases Capable of Generating Early Lassitude and Fatigue

| |
|---|
| Adrenal cortical insufficiency |
| Aldosteronism |
| Amyotrophic lateral sclerosis |
| Cirrhosis |
| Adult-onset diabetes mellitus |
| Hyperparathyroidism |
| Hyperthyroidism |
| Hypokalemia |
| Hypothyroidism |
| Systemic lupus erythematosus |
| Myasthenia gravis |
| Renal insufficiency |
| Anemia |
| Hypoxia |
| Congestive heart failure |

This intermingling of psychomotor symptomatology in general medical, neurologic, and psychiatric disease no doubt contributes to the impression in the psychosomatic literature of widespread association between medical and affective illness (for recent reviews see Hall, 1980; Rodin and Voshart, 1986). These nonspecific connections, however, make it much more difficult to identify heuristically important associations between affective and mediconeurologic disorders.

The converse of such a clinical dilemma is presented by the somatic symptoms that occur in many patients with psychiatric affective disorders. Dowling and Knox (1964) surveyed a group of patients with presumably primary depression and found that 43% of them experienced important somatic symptoms including abdominal discomfort, fatigue, nausea, headache, chest pain, and anorexia. More recent research has confirmed such observations and indicated that these vague somatic symptoms occur across all research diagnostic criteria depressive subtypes and are not confined to the endogenous subtype (Casper *et al.*, 1985). It seems likely that experienced clinicians are able to discriminate the psychiatric depressive symptomatology from the general medical with some reliability. Our goal in this chapter will be to make this process of discrimination as explicit as current research knowledge will allow.

There is a problem with regard to terminology with depressive syndromes that occur in the context of a general medical or neurologic disorder. What should they be called? It is currently fashionable to distinguish primary depression from secondary depression (Feighner *et al.*, 1972). Primary depression refers to a depressive syndrome that is not due to demonstrable physical illness and which occurs prior to the onset of another, nonaffective psychiatric syndrome. Secondary depression refers to a depressive syndrome that begins *after* the onset of another, nonaffective psychiatric illness. Should a depressive syndrome that begins after the onset of a medical or neurologic illness also be termed a secondary depression? Perhaps a tertiary depression? We would favor some such term. The *Diagnostic and Statistical Manual-III-Revised* (1987) requires the clinician to judge whether a depressive syndrome in the setting of medical illness is *caused by* or *secondary to* the medical illness. If so judged, the correct diagnosis becomes "organic mood disorder." If not, the syndrome is classified on axis I as one of the depressive disorders. We object to this classification and terminology because of the implication that an "organic" affective disorder is somehow qualitatively different from a "nonorganic" one. Such a distinction may apply, but we do not have the research base to be certain. In addition, we have been warned of the dangers inherent in judging "causality" between states of physical and emotional alteration. We do not know enough of psychosomatic connections to make these judgments. After this caveat we will not belabor the terminologic issues further.

We present in Table 5.2 what we call the "long list" of neurologic and

**Table 5.2**
Diseases Associated with Depressive Syndrome

| Drugs and toxins | Endocrine | Malignancy |
|---|---|---|
| *Antihypertensives*[a] | *Hypothyroidism* | *Brain tumor* |
| *Reserpine* | *Cushing's syndrome* | *Carcinoma of pancreas* |
| *Clonidine* | *Hyperthyroidism* | Lung carcinoma |
| *Propranolol* | *Diabetes mellitus* | Carcinomatosis |
| *Methyldopa* | Addison's disease | Lymphoma |
| *Guanethidine* | Hyperparathyroidism | Carcinoid syndrome |
| *Phenothiazines* | Hyperaldosteronism | |
| *Corticosteroids* | Acromegaly | |
| Digitalis | | |
| Sulfonamides | | |
| Ranitidine | | |
| Antituberculous agents | | |
| Antineoplastic agents | | |
| Hydralazine | | |
| Lidocaine | | |
| Bromides | | |
| Anticonvulsants | | |
| Narcotics | | |
| Narcotic antagonists | | |
| Indomethacin | | |
| Methysergide | | |
| Estrogens | | |
| Diphenoxylate | | |
| Dopamine agonists | | |
| Heavy metal intoxication | | |
| Phenylpropanolamine | | |
| **Metabolic** | **Epilepsy** | **Neurodegenerative** |
| *Anemia* | Partial complex | *Parkinson's disease* |
| *Renal failure* | | *Alzheimer's disease* |
| $B_{12}$ deficiency | | Blindness |
| Folate deficiency | | Deafness |
| Hepatic failure | | Pick's disease |
| Amyloidosis | | Huntington's disease |
| Gout | | |
| Anoxia | | |
| | **Immunologic** | **Infection** |
| | Systemic lupus erythematosus | *Neurosyphilis* |
| | *Multiple sclerosis* | Hepatitis |
| | Rheumatoid arthritis | Herpes simplex |
| | Migraine | AIDS |
| | Periarteritis nodosa | *Epstein-Barr virus* |
| | Sarcoidosis | Tuberculosis |

(*continued*)

**Table 5.2** *(Continued)*

| | |
|---|---|
| | Giant-cell arteritis<br>Regional enteritis<br>Ulcerative colitis |
| Atherosclerotic | |
| Stroke | |

[a]Italicized entities are discussed in the text.

general medical diseases that have been reported to occur in association with the depressive syndrome. The problem with tables such as this is that the human brain, unlike an analog computer, cannot use them very well. People are forever memorizing and forgetting such tables or else carrying lists around that never quite match the clinical situation at hand. We propose several partial solutions to this problem, each of which (we hope) derives from preferred modes of human CNS function (i.e., is "user-friendly"). First, we have organized this table as well as the comprehensive tables in the other chapters, according to the following mnemonic:

| D | E | $M^2$ | E | N | T | $I^2$ | A |
|---|---|---|---|---|---|---|---|
| Drugs and toxins | Endocrine | Malignancy metabolic | Epilepsy | Neuro-degenerative | Trauma | Immunologic infection | Athero-sclerotic |

This mnemonic is not perfect. For example, it is somewhat unclear where "migraine" should go (we have picked the immunologic section in deference to Norman Geschwind). And of course, it is possible to forget the mnemonic, which we have done on occasion. Still, this tool proves useful for those relatively rare clinical situations in which one is "stuck" and wishes to review possible diagnostic categories in a systematic fashion. We will discuss the individual syndromes in this chapter according to this DEMENTIA organization.

We believe that experienced clinicians are relatively rarely stuck in diagnostic dilemmas because of their ability to recognize several basic *patterns* within various categories of behavioral pathology. Our brain is far superior to analog computers in recognizing patterns, in contradistinction to our clumsiness at remembering lists. Moreover, the number of patterns we tend to recognize within a category such as "depressive spectrum disorder" is not large. No one is clinically familiar with all the diseases in Table 5.2. Our goal in this chapter, as in the subsequent ones, will be to select those general medical and neurologic diseases that are *most likely* to present intermingled with depressive symptomatology and to discuss those diseases from the perspective of their clinical and laboratory *patterns*. Those general medical diseases or syndromes that we will discuss in some detail are italicized in Table 5.2.

## DRUGS AND TOXINS

A 29-year-old man is given haloperidol for Tourette's syndrome. At a dosage of 0.5 mg BID, he notices some improvement in vocal and motor tics. When the dosage reaches 1 mg BID, he suddenly develops spontaneous weeping spells and a sense of despondency. The dosage is reduced back to 0.5 mg BID, and the dysphoric symptoms resolve.

### Background

There is an extensive and controversial research literature concerning alterations in monoamine metabolism that occur in depressive disorders (for recent reviews see Mann *et al.*, 1985; Lake and Ziegler, 1985; Post and Ballenger, 1984). Older studies associated clinical depressive disorders with evidence of CNS catecholamine or indoleamine depletion, but more recent research has failed to confirm such deficits. Receptor sensitivity appears to be an important factor, as are clinical distinctions such as bipolar versus unipolar depressive states. Generalizations are dangerous, except to say that monoamine metabolism within CNS is involved in some important way with affective sensation and display. The major monoamines are depicted in Fig. 5.1.

A useful clinical rule in evaluating depressive episodes for patients taking nonpsychiatric medications is the following:

---

*Clinical Rule 5.1:* Drugs that block, release, up-regulate, down-regulate, or otherwise modify catecholamine or indoleamine systems are capable of inducing depression.

---

### Antihypertensive Drugs

As Table 5.2 indicates, most of the drugs that are given to reduce blood pressure have been reported at one time or another to be associated with depressive symptoms. Reserpine, a Rauwolfia alkaloid, has been the most carefully studied drug in this regard (for reviews see Goodwin and Bunney, 1971; Quetsch *et al.*, 1959). This drug depletes both serotonin and catecholamines from storage sites in brain and peripheral nerve and has been associated with varying rates of depressive side effects. When Goodwin and Bunney (1971) reviewed these reports, however, they felt that the general psychomotor slowing and parkinsonism produced by the drug had often been confounded with

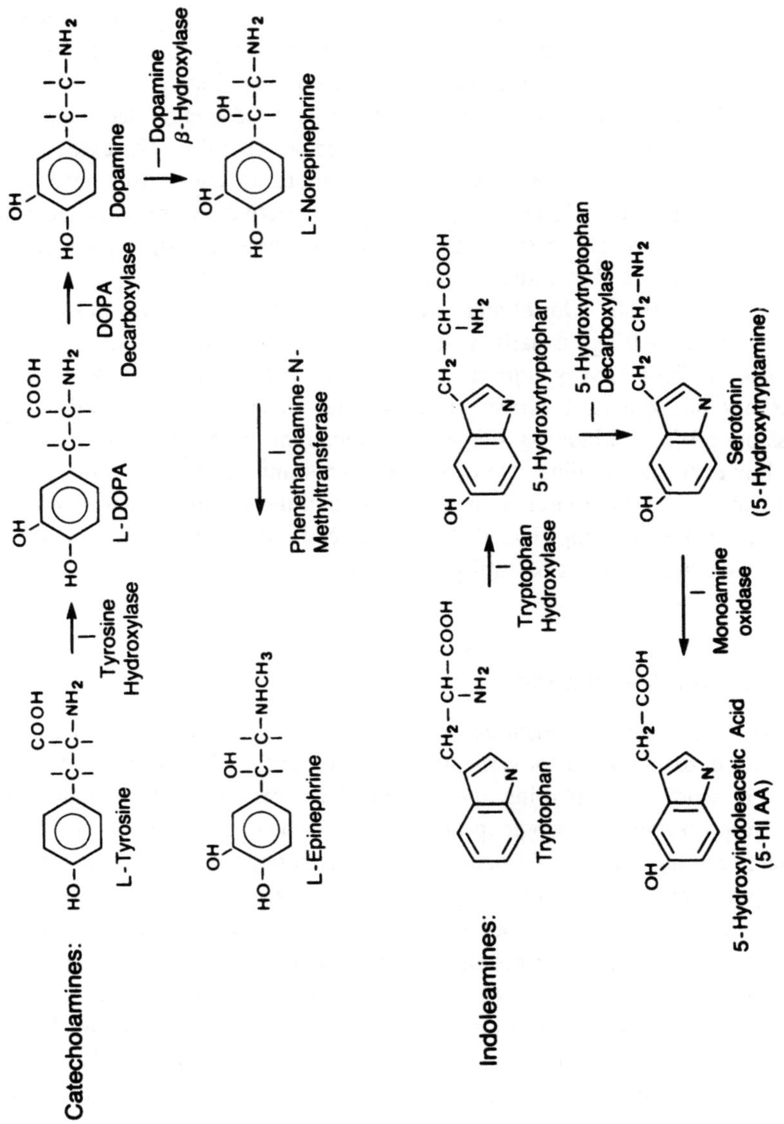


**Figure 5.1.** CNS monoamines.

depressive symptoms. They concluded that the overall rate of "true" depressions for persons taking reserpine was perhaps in the range of 5%. Most of these depressive episodes occurred at dosages greater than 0.5 mg day, and in many cases the individuals seemed *predisposed* to an affective disorder as evidenced by a history of previous affective episodes. It is worth remembering that some of the depressive events described in these reports occurred several months to 1 or 2 years after the start of drug administration.

The other antihypertensive drugs in Table 5.2 are adrenergic depleters which work by various mechanisms, either centrally or peripherally. The evidence for an association with dysphoric side effects is more anecdotal for these drugs than it is for reserpine. There are open and retrospective reports indicating that 10–30% of patients taking propranolol or methyldopa develop significant depressive side effects, but blinded controlled studies are lacking (Waal, 1967; Pritchard *et al.*, 1968). Our clinical experience with this issue has mostly been in the inpatient setting, usually with multisystem sick individuals who have multifactorial depressive syndromes. Manipulating the antihypertensive medications has not generally proved a spectacular success in ameliorating their depressions. We continue to suggest modifications of antihypertensive regimens, however, as an adjunct to other antidepressant strategies. At the present time it appears that the diuretics, hydralazine, and the calcium channel blockers are relatively free of drug-related dysphoria, and we prefer to treat depressed patients with these classes of antihypertensives.

## Antipsychotic Medications

The dopaminergic transmitter systems within the CNS have been more implicated in disorders of movement and psychosis than in disorders of mood. Still, it is worth remembering that L-dopa has been reported to have antidepressant properties in a subgroup of depressed patients (Goodwin *et al.*, 1970), and there are case reports of "neuroleptic-induced depression" in patients taking antipsychotic drugs (Caine and Polinsky, 1979). We have seen this phenomenon in clinical practice and suspect that it is underreported. As with reserpine, the dysphoria has a dosage threshold and tends to appear as the drug is being increased. The dysphoria may not immediately resolve after a dosage reduction, which is sometimes not possible with psychotic patients. We believe this phenomenon to be more common with the high-potency antipsychotics such as haloperidol, but we do not have data to support this clinical impression. Patients can be switched to low-potency agents such as thioridazine, and antidepressants can be added to the regimen when drug-related depressive symptoms appear.

## Corticosteroids

There is an interesting but poorly understood phenomenon with regard to corticosteroids and affect. When exogenous steroids are given acutely, one typically sees psychomotor acceleration and mood elevation (see Chapter 6). In Cushing's disease and Cushing's syndrome, however, where the patient must adjust to chronically elevated levels of steroid hormones, *depression* and *dysphoric* symptoms are by far the more common. Depressive symptomatology may also emerge during long-term exogenous corticosteroid administration or during the tapering phase of an acute pharmacologic course of these drugs. For a full discussion of these issues see Shader's review (1972).

## Other Medications

A variety of other medications have been reported in association with the depressive syndrome, and an even more comprehensive list is discussed in Shader's book (1972). Most of the literature to substantiate these associations is anecdotal. We would not say that in any individual patient, any individual drug from digitalis to cyclophosphamide might not be capable of precipitating a dysphoric state—such individualized judgments remain the clinician's burden. What we would say is that for most of these other drugs there is no systematic understanding of such an association, no theoretic reason by which to expect it, and few empirical data by which to confirm it.

# ENDOCRINE DISEASE AND DEPRESSION

## Hypothyroidism

A 26-year-old woman with dysthymia has proved refractory to psychotherapy and tricyclics. A second opinion is requested. On interview, she is humorless, with downcast facies and dysphoria. On physical examination she appears pale and has generalized psychomotor slowing. Heart rate is 60 and regular. Reflexes are symmetric, but slow to relax. Serum $T_4$ is 4.0; $T_3$ RU is 20%; TSH is 12.0.

### Background

It is useful for psychiatrists to consider hypothyroidism to be a *clinical* condition produced by a deficiency of circulating thyroid hormones ($T_3$, $T_4$). Diseases that affect the thyroid gland itself may produce hypothyroidism, as may diseases that affect higher regulatory centers, such as anterior pituitary and

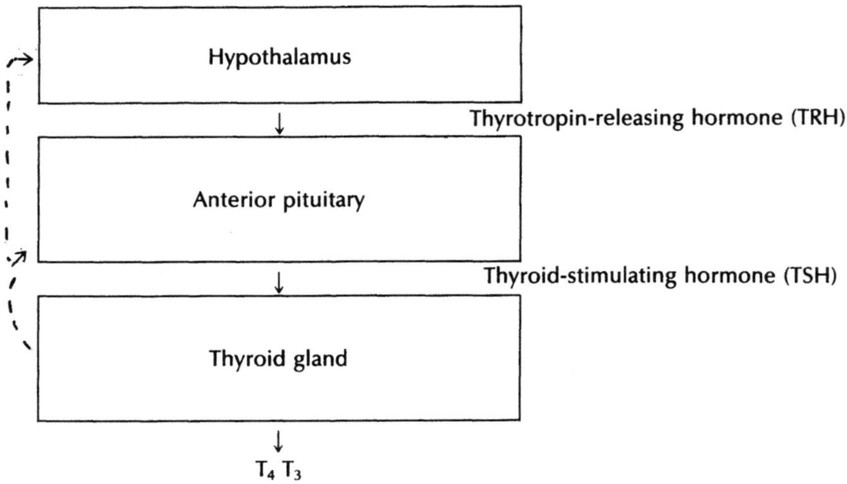


**Figure 5.2.** Schema of regulatory relationships in hypothyroidism.

hypothalamus. It is worthwhile to remember a simplified schema of these regulatory relationships, with their feedback loops (Fig. 5.2).

An understanding of the negative feedback loops depicted by the dotted lines in Fig. 5.2 is important in the interpretation of much of the current literature concerning relationships between thyroid function and depression. Diseases of the thyroid gland itself, such as primary idiopathic hypothyroidism or hypothyroidism secondary to chronic thyroiditis (Hashimoto's disease), are associated with low levels of circulating thyroid hormones but elevated circulating TRH and TSH. When exogenous TRH or TRH-like peptides such as Protirelin are administered to such patients, an *exaggerated* TSH response occurs. Diseases of anterior pituitary and hypothalamus may also produce hypothyroidism, but in these patients exogenous TRH administration may result in a *blunted* rise in TSH. As we shall see, there is evidence that clinical depression may be seen with both sorts of thyroid dysfunction.

Gold and co-workers have published a series of studies indicating that 8–15% of patients admitted to their hospital with depression demonstrate abnormalities on thyroid function tests (Gold, 1981a,b, 1982). The thyroid function tests included $T_3$RU, $T_4$, TSH, and TRH (Protirelin) stimulation. They classified 20 patients (8%) from this group as hypothyroid, but in ten of these patients the only evidence for hypothyroidism was an exaggerated TSH response to Protirelin injection. They suggest the following classification of hypothyroidism:

| | | | | |
|---|---|---|---|---|
| Overt: | $T_3$RU ↓ | $T_4$ ↓ | TSH ↑ | Clinical signs(+) |
| Mild: | $T_3$RU normal | $T_4$ normal | TSH ↑ | Isolated clinical signs (+) |
| Subclinical: | All tests normal except TRH stimulation. Clinical examination normal. | | | |

In a quite different line of investigation, however, a series of studies has indicated that as many as 25% of depressed patients may demonstrate *blunting* of TSH rise after TRH stimulation (for review see Loosen and Prange, 1982). In this review, a blunted response was defined as a peak TSH rise less than 5 $\mu$U/ml. There is evidence that this blunting may be somewhat nonspecific, appearing also in anorexia, alcoholism, and mania.

We are not doubting the clinical association between mild hypothyroidism and depressive syndromes. Indeed, this is one of the best-studied, specific associations between medical and behavioral syndromes. Perhaps as many as 40% of patients with hypothyroidism demonstrate features of depression, apathy, psychomotor slowing, and amnesia (Loosen and Prange, 1984). But our bias in this book remains one of relying on *clinical* data, obtained during the interview and examination. Therefore, we remain skeptical toward the "subclinical" hypothyroid group among depressed patients. Treatment data are not yet available concerning the administration of thyroid hormone to these patients. Moreover, there is evidence that transient fluctuation in thyroid indices occurs among psychiatric patients, even as it does among medical patients under the stress of systemic illness (Cohen and Swigar, 1979). For the present, we insist on an elevated TSH (preferably *after* the first 2 weeks of an inpatient stay) before initiating thyroid hormone replacement, and we strongly prefer to see at least one clinical sign or symptom of hypothyroidism beyond the depression itself.

## Demographics

A sense of rough demographic trends concerning a syndrome such as hypothyroidism is essential in conferring the sort of "reasonable probability" clinical suspicion that makes accurate diagnosis and avoids wasteful diagnostic tests. Every known disease is "common" within some delimited patient population. Without this sense, the appropriate clinical history is omitted, and the clinical signs are missed, because in this interaction with the patient:

---

*Clinical Rule 5.2:* Believing is seeing in the psychiatric interview and examination. If you don't think of it, you won't find it.

*Cautionary Lemma 5.2a:* Even a blind squirrel finds an occasional acorn.

---

Hypothyroidism in adults is predominantly a disease of women, with female:male ratios as high as 7:1 for many etiologies. The most common hypothyroid syndrome is probably iatrogenic, post-$^{131}$I, or surgical ablation in treatment of Graves' disease. Hypothyroidism secondary to chronic thyroiditis (Hashimoto's disease) may be associated with goiter. Both of these hypothyroid syndromes most commonly appear during the third and fourth decades. An autoimmune form of hypothyroidism associated with glandular atrophy and antithyroid antibodies is more common among elderly women (Bonnyns *et al.*, 1982).

Hypothyroidism on an autoimmune basis is also associated with other autoimmune diseases, such as $B_{12}$ deficiency, systemic lupus erythematosus, or myasthenia gravis. There are other causes of hypothyroidism, but we hope that the following features can "clue" the clinician to be alert for most of them.

## Clinical History

Important clues to be listened for during the clinical history include:

1. Family history. Some of the immune-based hypothyroid syndromes are mediated by specific HLA haplotypes. Have female relatives had thyroid difficulties?
2. Cold intolerance. Does the patient wear sweaters or jackets when others feel warm? Is this a change?
3. Constipation. Especially important if coinciding in time with the depressive symptoms.
4. Menorrhagia. Has there been a change toward profuse or prolonged menstrual periods?
5. Hair change, skin change, appetite change. These questions have not been useful in our experience, because many depressed patients will accede to them.

## Psychotropic Drug Interactions

**Lithium.** Lithium has a direct antithyroid effect at the level of the gland itself and is capable of producing both subclinical and overt hypothyroidism (Calabrese *et al.*, 1985; Smigan *et al.*, 1984). There may be an additional immunoregulatory factor in lithium's antithyroid action. Patients typically develop elevated TSH, low $T_4$, low free $T_4$, and clinical signs or symptoms. Antithyroid antibodies may also appear in such patients.

**Phenytoin.** Phenytoin competes with $T_4$ for binding sites on thyroxine-binding globulin, producing an artifactually depressed total $T_4$ with a normal free $T_4$. These patients are not clinically hypothyroid.

## Mental Status Examination

Hypothyroid patients complain of difficulty in concentration, and they demonstrate poor performance in tasks of serial performance (Whybrow, 1969). These abnormalities are reversible with treatment.

## General Medical Examination

Vital Signs. Bradycardia.

Skin. Thickening; pale; pretibial myxedema, which is a nonpitting, doughy, thickening of subcutaneous tissue in pretibial or other regions.

GI. Adynamic ileus or decreased bowel sounds may be present.

Hair. May appear dry, and areas of new hair loss may be evident.

## Neurologic Examination

Motor. Generalized psychomotor slowing; poor performance on rapid alternating movements.

Reflexes. "Hung-up" quality of reflexes (i.e., slow relaxation phase).

Cranial Nerves. Limited oculomotor excursion or proptosis may be present in patients with Graves' ophthalmopathy. Hoarseness may be an early sign.

## Laboratory and Imaging

*Note:* U.S. medical journals are embarking on a 2-year period of conversion in scientific units of measurement to Système International (SI) units. The normal ranges in this book will be given both in conventional and the new SI units (normal ranges taken from *JAMA* Editorial 1986) (see Table 5.3).

### TRH Stimulation Test (from Gold, 1981a)

| | Time(min): 0 | 15 | 30 | 45 | 60 | 90 |
|---|---|---|---|---|---|---|
| Inject 500 μg Protirelin IV over 30 sec | Baseline TSH | TSH | TSH | TSH | TSH | TSH |

**Table 5.3**
Normal Ranges for Selected Thyroid Tests

| Test | Fluid | Current normal range | SI reference interval | Comment |
|---|---|---|---|---|
| $T_4$ (thyroxine) | Serum | 4–11 μg/dl | 51–142 nmole/liter | |
| $T_4$ free | Serum | 0.8–2.8 ng/dl | 10–36 pmole/liter | |
| $T_3$ (triiodothyronine) | Serum | 75–220 ng/dl | 1.2–3.4 nmole/liter | |
| $T_3$ resin uptake | Serum | 25–35% | 0.25–0.35 | An indirect measure of the number of binding sites available for $T_3$. Typically $T_3$ RU is decreased in hypothyroidism |
| TSH | Serum | 2–11 μU/ml | 2–11 mU/ml | |

The normal rise in TSH should exceed 5 μU/ml but should be less than 30 μU/ml.

Ultrasound. To be done when thyroid nodule is palpated; separates cystic from solid nodules.

Thyroid Scans. $^{131}I$ uptake. Rates of tracer iodide accumulation in the thyroid gland can be measured over periods of time up to 24 hr. The saturation of Western diets with iodide makes this test less useful in diagnostic evaluation of hypothyroidism. The test is more useful in the evaluation of hyperthyroidism. $^{99m}Tc$ pertechnetate imaging scan may help to distinguish functioning thyroid tissue. See Fig. 5.3.

Needle Biopsy. For evaluation of nodules. Endocrine consultation is appropriate by this point.

## Hyperthyroidism

We present our detailed clinical profile of hyperthyroidism in Chapter 7, since this endocrine dysfunction more typically presents with symptoms of anxiety and nervousness. Clinicians are reminded, however, of the syndrome termed "apathetic thyrotoxicosis," which may mimic a major depressive episode (Thomas *et al.*, 1970; Taylor, 1975). These patients tend to be elderly and to

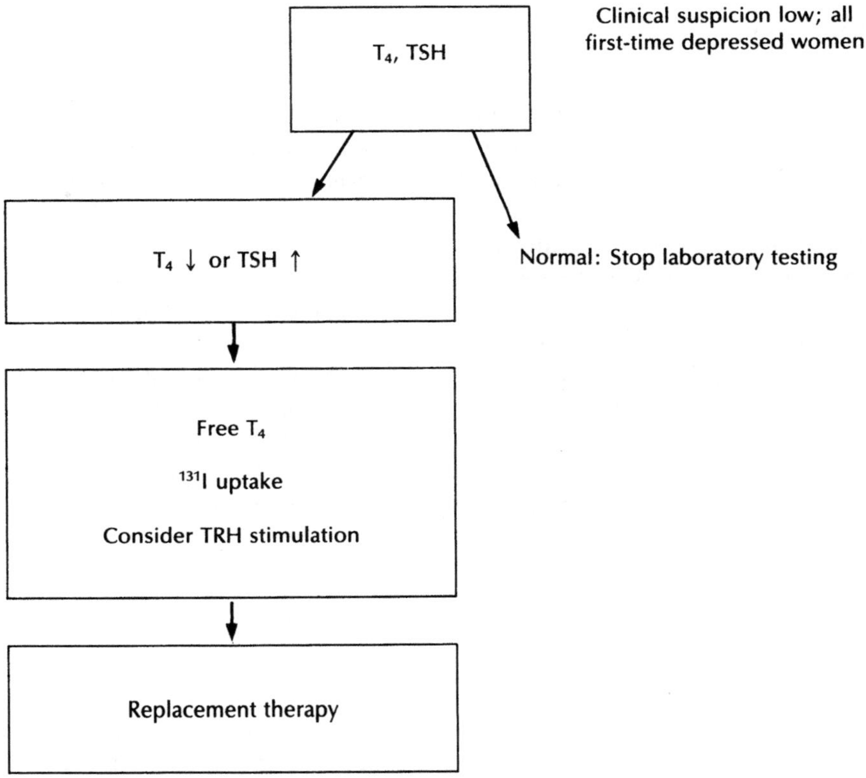


**Figure 5.3.** Overview of laboratory approach to suspected hypothyroidism.

demonstrate blepharoptosis and multinodular goiter on physical examination. Atrial fibrillation is common and has proved a useful clinical clue in our experience. On neurologic examination, most of such patients demonstrate proximal muscle wasting, especially within hip girdle musculature, and a fine postural tremor, distal more than proximal.

## Cushing's Syndrome

A 26-year-old woman has developed an atypical depressive disorder, characterized by histrionic weeping, mental dullness, instability, and emotional lability. Since she has significant suicidal potential, she is admitted to the psychiatry service for evaluation and treatment. The peer review protocol for depressed patients at this hospital includes a dexamethasone suppression test, which demonstrates reassuring "escape" (i.e., serum cortisol $>5$ $\mu$g/DL) on the 5:00 PM level. On physical examination she demonstrates *galactorrhea*.

## Background

Reasonable clinical evidence now exists for a specific endocrine–psychiatric connection between hypercortisolism and depression. Patients with Cushing's disease or Cushing's syndrome demonstrate depressive features with incidence rates approaching 60%, a rate significantly higher than that in patients with nonbasophilic pituitary tumors (Michael and Gibbons, 1963; Kelly *et al.*, 1983). In many cases, the affective disorder may appear prior to, or simultaneous with, diagnosis of the endocrine disorder (Hudson *et al.*, 1987). And, of course, every psychiatrist and quality control auditor knows that approximately two-thirds of psychiatric patients with major depressive episodes demonstrate evidence of Cushing's syndrome on the 1-mg dexamethasone suppression test (Zimmerman *et al.*, 1986). We do not have good studies concerning the number of nonaffective Cushing's syndrome and Cushing's disease patients who are hidden within this 66% of depressed patients. And herein lies an important clinical diagnostic opportunity for psychiatrists, because of our clinical rule 5.3.

---

*Clinical Rule 5.3:* An abnormal DST indicates the presence of Cushing's syndrome. It does not indicate the cause of that syndrome.

---

Normally, cortisol is secreted from the adrenal cortex under the trophic influence of ACTH (adrenocorticotrophic hormone) from the anterior pituitary. This secretion does not occur at a steady rate, but in small bursts with an overall diurnal rhythm such that serum cortisol levels tend to be highest in the early morning and lowest in the evening. "Cushing's syndrome" refers to the clinical condition in which the overall 24-hr cortisol secretion is abnormally increased. In general, the secretion pattern remains episodic, but the circadian rhythm is abolished. Depression is one of several causes of Cushing's syndrome. Table 5.4 presents a classification of such causes.

**Table 5.4**
Causes of Cushing's Syndrome

| |
|---|
| Cushing's syndrome secondary to increased ACTH production |
| Pituitary–hypothalamic dysfunction possibly related to increased corticotropin-releasing factor (CRF) release. Example: depression |
| Pituitary ACTH producing adenoma (Cushing's disease) |
| Ectopic ACTH or ACTH-like production. Example: bronchogenic carcinoma |
| Cushing's syndrome secondary to autonomous adrenal cortex production of cortisol |
| Adrenal nodular hyperplasia |
| Adrenal neoplasia |

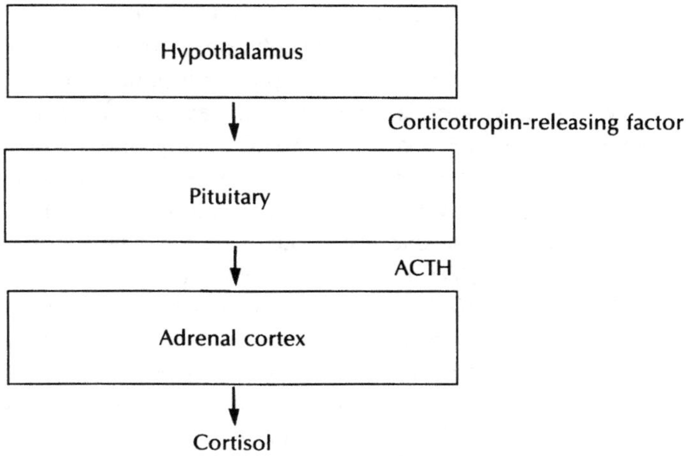


**Figure 5.4.** Brain mechanism of cortisol secretion.

If one keeps in mind a simplistic image of the way in which the brain controls cortisol secretion (Fig. 5.4), one can see that there are only a couple of ways in which the system can go wrong on the hypersecretion side. The hypothalamus may oversecrete CRF or secrete it in an abnormal pattern. This is the level of the cortisol axis we understand the least, but it is probably here that the dysfunction of depression occurs. The pituitary may oversecrete ACTH. This is usually produced by a basophilic adenoma, and it is this syndrome alone that should be termed Cushing's disease. These tumors tend to be small. ACTH or ACTH-like peptides may also be produced by neoplastic cells elsewhere in the body. This is termed ectopic ACTH secretion, and it is most commonly associated with carcinoma of the lung but can also be seen in pancreatic carcinoma and thymoma. In the cases of both pituitary and nonpituitary neoplastic secretion of ACTH, the patient demonstrates elevated serum cortisol *as well as* elevated serum ACTH. Cortisol may also be abnormally hypersecreted by the adrenal cortex itself. This can occur in the setting of bilateral adrenal hyperplasia or carcinoma of the adrenal cortex. In these syndromes, measures of serum cortisol are elevated, but ACTH is *depressed* by feedback inhibition. Unfortunately, it does not appear that serum ACTH levels may be used to distinguish Cushing's syndrome due to depression from Cushing's syndrome due to neoplastic ACTH secretion. For a recent review of these diagnostic issues see Carpenter (1986).

The psychiatrist's core diagnostic issue remains the separation of affective Cushing's syndrome from the other forms of Cushing's syndrome. Fortunately or unfortunately for psychiatric clinicians, recent advances in neuroendocrine laboratory testing have not provided much help with this issue. Two tests do show promise for making this distinction. The best test at present seems to be the cortisol response to insulin-induced hypoglycemia (Aron *et al.*, 1981). With a running IV and glucose readily available, regular insulin is injected IV in 2- to 4-unit doses. Plasma glucose is followed with Dextrostix until it is below 40 mg/dl. Under these conditions, plasma cortisol usually rises to a level above 20 $\mu$g/dl. In the depressive syndrome this response can be expected, but in Cushing's syndrome from other causes, the elevated baseline cortisol does not tend to increase further. A second test, which remains experimental, involves measurement of plasma ACTH response to IV corticotropin-releasing hormone (Gold *et al.*, 1986). Depressed patients may demonstrate an attenuated plasma ACTH response to a CRF infusion in contrast with patients who have Cushing's disease, who demonstrate ACTH hyperresponsiveness.

The diagnostic feature upon which psychiatric clinicians must rely in the differential assessment of Cushing's syndrome is that the affective patients do not become cushingoid. That is, these patients demonstrate depression and failure to suppress on low-dose (and sometimes on high-dose) dexamethasone suppression tests, but they do not demonstrate the physical stigmata of Cushing's syndrome from other etiologies. The reason for this is not understood. We can return now to our opening vignette in this section of the 26-year-old woman with depression and galactorrhea. She *probably* has Cushing's disease, because she demonstrates at least one cushingoid feature. She deserves a careful evaluation for causes of Cushing's syndrome other than depression.

## Demographics

The incidence of pituitary ACTH-producing adenomas in women is three times the incidence in men. The most frequent age of onset is the third or fourth decade. The syndromes of ectopic ACTH production are rarer and parallel the demographics of the tumors that produce them (i.e., bronchogenic and pancreatic carcinomas). At the present time, middle-aged and older men with heavy smoking histories would experience higher risk for such syndromes.

## Clinical History

The following historical features may be clues to the presence of nonaffective Cushing's syndrome. As in all clinical history taking with psychiatric patients, the value of these features rises considerably if they are *volunteered* by the patient, as opposed to elicitation by direct questioning.

**Muscle Weakness and Fatigability.** Chronically high levels of glucocorticosteroids can produce a myopathy and weakness. Complaints of proximal muscle weakness (i.e., stair climbing, hair combing) are more suspicious than those of distal weakness.

History of recent onset *osteporosis:* Has there been a spontaneous fracture or compression fracture?

Easy *bruisability,* especially if described as something new.

Galactorrhea. If an anterior pituitary microadenoma has grown sufficiently to encroach upon prolactin-secreting cells, the inhibitory effect of this hormone upon lactation can be impaired.

Diabetes Mellitus. The glucocorticosteroids are gluconeogenic, and cushingoid patients who are genetically or physiologically predisposed may develop overt diabetes.

Hypertension. The glucocorticoid excess of Cushing's syndrome includes some mineralocorticoid effect as well, predisposing to hypertension.

Amenorrhea. May occur in Cushing's syndrome.

## Psychotropic Drug Interactions

Nonspecific.

## Mental Status Examination

Cognition. Patients with Cushing's syndrome demonstrate deficits on neuropsychological tests measuring visuospatial and visuomemory functions (Whelan *et al.*, 1980). Language functions tend to be preserved. Starkman and colleagues have shown that bedside tests of verbal recall (recall of three cities) and of concentration and attention (serial 7 subtraction) correlate quite well with the results of more extensive neuropsychological testing (Starkman *et al.*, 1986). These deficits are reversible with treatment of the syndrome.

Depression. If it is comprehensible to consider the group of patients who have "depressed nonaffective Cushing's syndrome," it is worth remarking that clinical observers have mentioned *atypical* qualities of the depression (Trethowan and Cobb, 1952). In contrast with the more typically endogenous quality of DST nonsuppressors among psychiatric patients, these Cushing's syndrome patients tend to display features of dullness, irritability, histrionicity, and true emotional lability.

## General Medical Examination

Vital Signs. Hypertension?

Skin. Reddish or purplish abdominal striae may appear secondary to weakening and rupture of collagenous fibers in the dermis. If increased production of androgenic steroids also occurs, hirsutism and acne may appear. Facial flushing is sometimes seen.

Musculoskeletal. A characteristic redistribution of fat stores occurs in Cushing's syndrome in a centripetal manner. "Moon" facies may develop as a result, as well as the interscapular "buffalo hump."

## Neurological Examination

After sustained Cushing's syndrome, myopathic pattern weakness (i.e., proximal weaker than distal) may develop along with proximal muscle atrophy. Such weakness is typically not profound but would be graded from 4 to 5 on the 0-to-5 scale.

## Laboratory and Imaging

Screening Tests. Hypokalemia and increased serum cholesterol may be noted on incidental, screening chemistries. See Table 5.5 and Fig. 5.5.

**Table 5.5**
Neuroendocrine, Suppression, and Stimulation Tests

| Test | Fluid | Normal range | Comment |
|---|---|---|---|
| Neuroendocrine tests | | | |
| ACTH | Plasma | 20–100 pg/ml (4–22 pmole/liter) | |
| Cortisol 8 AM | Serum | 4–19 μg/dl (110–520 mmole/liter) | |
| 6 PM | Serum | 2–15 μg/dl (50–410 nmole/liter) | |
| Midnight | Serum | <5 μg/dl (<140 nmole/liter) | |
| Cortisol | 24-hr urine | 10–110 μg/24 hr (30–300 nmole) | Probably the best screening test. Not weight-dependent |
| 17-Hydroxysteroids | 24-hr urine | | |
| Female | | 2–8 mg/24 hr (5–25 μmole/day) | |
| Male | | 3–10 mg/24 hr (10–30 μmole/day) | |

*(continued)*

**Table 5.5** *(Continued)*

| | | | |
|---|---|---|---|
| 17-Ketosteroids | 24-hr urine | | |
| Female | | 6–17 mg/24 hr (20–60 μmole/day) | |
| Male | | 6–20 mg/24 hr (20–70 μmole/day) | |
| Suppression tests | | | |
| Screening dexamethasone suppression tests | | | |
| Day 1: Give 1 mg dexamethasone PO at 11:00 PM<br>Day 2: Check 6:00 PM and midnight serum cortisol | | | Both cortisol levels should suppress to <5 μg/dl |
| Standard dexamethasone suppression tests | | | |
| Days 1 and 2: Give dexamethasone 0.5 mg PO every 6 hr<br>Day 3: 24-hr urine for free cortisol and 17-hydroxysteroids | | | 24-hr 17-hydroxysteroid should suppress to <3 mg; 24-hr urinary free cortisol should suppress to <30 μg; serum cortisol levels should suppress as for screening test |
| High-dose dexamethasone suppression test | | | |
| Days 1 and 2: 2 mg dexamethasone PO every 6 hr<br>Day 3: As for standard test | | | 10–15% of patients with Cushing's disease and most patients with ectopic ACTH production fail to suppress on this test |
| Stimulation test | | | |
| Metyrapone stimulation (Spiger *et al.*, 1975) | | | |
| Day 1: 3 g metyrapone PO HS<br>Day 2: Measure plasma cortisol and 11-deoxycortisol levels | | | Increased production of compound S (11-deoxycortisol) to level of 10 μg/dl, with fall of serum cortisol below 7 μg/ml |
| Imaging | | | |
| CT scan of sella turcica | | | Remains normal in approximately 50% of patients known to have microadenoma |
| CT of adrenals | | | May recognize adrenal tumors to 1 cm diameter |

## Addison's Disease

Even as there is a puzzling inverse relationship between the affective disturbances that tend to be seen with exogenous as opposed to endogenous increased levels of corticosteroid excess, so we must remark that Addison's disease has been associated with depressive episodes as well as Cushing's disease.

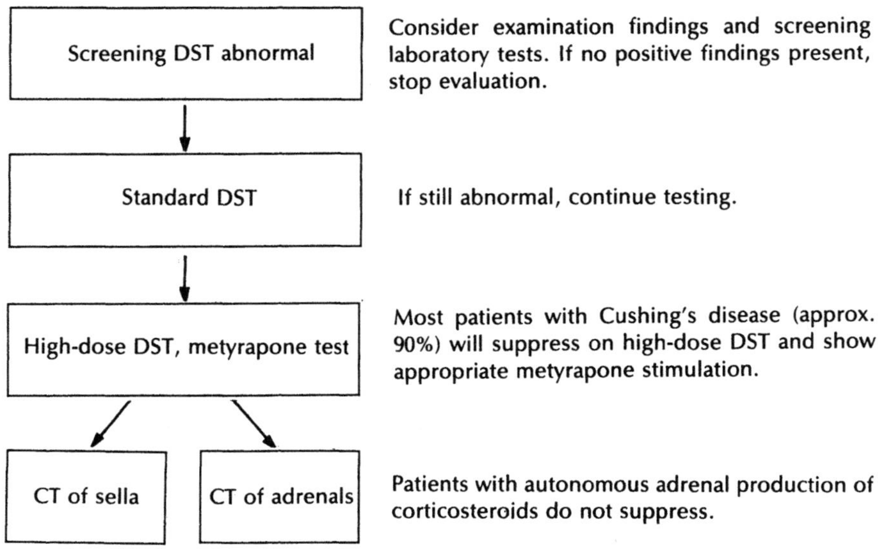


**Figure 5.5.** Overview of laboratory approach to Cushing's syndrome.

Addison's disease is much less common than Cushing's disease or syndrome among psychiatric patients, so we will not profile this medical disease in detail. Whybrow and Horwitz (1976), in their review of psychological syndromes associated with endocrine disturbance, reported that approximately 16% of addisonian patients can be expected to have disturbed cognition, and 13% have features of depression with some overlap between groups. It appears that very few, if any, of such patients turn up "hidden" within psychiatric populations. Case reports of Addison's disease masquerading as agitated depression are still publishable (Varadaraj and Cooper, 1986). Important clinical features of such patients include hypotension, hyperpigmentation, weakness without atrophy, elevated serum potassium, and hypoglycemia.

## Hyperparathyroidism

There is no evidence that primary or secondary hyperparathyroidism occurs with any significant frequency among psychiatric patient populations. Such a phenomenon may still generate a case report (Borer and Bhanof, 1985). In our combined experience we have seen one such person—an elderly woman who presented with dysphoric and paranoid features but who demonstrated a major element of confusion on her mental status examination. In the few series available in the literature concerning mental status changes associated with hyperparathyroidism, psychomotor slowing, depression, memory disturbance, and delirium tend to predominate (Karpati and Frame, 1964; Petersen, 1968; Gatewood *et al.*, 1975). This diagnosis occurs to clinicians when they look at the SMA-12 page in the laboratory reports, not when they look at the patient. The pattern to watch for on the SMA-12 is: elevated calcium; low-normal or subnormal phosphorus; mildly elevated alkaline phosphatase. When this pattern appears, the clinician should repeat the tests, order a bone survey for subcortical resorption of bone, and ask for an endocrine consultation.

## Diabetes Mellitus

Many of the large surveys of medical illness reviewed in Chapter 2 include diabetes mellitus as a "cause" of mental status abnormalities. We believe that such a hypothesis requires additional research before it is accepted. Our experience has been that glucose intolerance, although not uncommon when of a mild degree, rarely provides the therapeutic key to a behavioral disorder. Sometimes the psychotropic drugs prescribed for a psychiatric patient contribute to the glucose intolerance. The clinician usually sees an elevated glucose upon an inpatient's SMA-6, and he must consider the implications while concurrently treating the psychiatric disorder.

Beresford and colleagues (1985) have reported a prevalence rate of 9% among psychiatric outpatients for elevated serum glucose with concomitant urinary glucose or ketones. It is important to remember that a random glucose, such as might appear on an inpatient's SMA-6, is of value only to alert the clinician. A variety of clinical states, including recent meals, infection, and agitation, may elevate the serum glucose. For psychiatric inpatients, the best course is to wait a few days, allowing the behavior to settle, and then to perform a glucose tolerance test (National Diabetes Data Group, 1979).

### OGTT

At time 0, fasting plasma glucose. Give 75 g glucose PO (for nonpregnant adults). At 30, 60, 90, and 120 min, plasma glucoses.

### Criteria for Diabetes Mellitus in Nonpregnant Adults

1. Elevated FBS on more than one occasion. Venous plasma ≥ 140 mg/dl (7.8 mmole/liter); venous whole blood ≥ 120 mg/dl (6.7 mmole/liter); capillary whole blood ≥ 120 mg/dl (6.7 mmole/liter).
2. On OGTT the 2-hr sample *and* one other sample must meet these criteria: venous plasma glucose ≥ 200 mg/dl (11.1 mmole/liter); venous whole blood glucose ≥ 180 mg/dl (10.0 mmole/liter); capillary whole blood glucose ≥ 200 mg/dl.
3. Criteria for impaired glucose tolerance (an intermediate state): (a) FBS

normal; (b) one of the 30-, 60-, or 90-min OGTT values must be elevated; (c) the OGTT 120-min value must be: (a) venous plasma glucose 140–200 mg/dl; (b) venous whole blood glucose 120–180 mg/dl; (c) capillary glucose 140–200 mg/dl.

### Psychotropic Drug Interactions

Drugs that have been reported to contribute to impaired glucose tolerance: chlorprothixene, haloperidol, $LiCO_3$, phenothiazines, tricyclic antidepressants. Drugs that may interfere with laboratory tests for glucose: isocarboxazid (decreased glucose value when measured by glucose oxidase method), nitrazepam (same effect).

# IMMUNOLOGICAL DISEASE AND DEPRESSION

## Collagen Vascular Diseases

There is substantial literature linking CNS systemic lupus erythematosus with a variety of behavioral syndromes, including depressive affective disorders. Many of these reports suggest that an atypical psychosis may be commonly encountered in such patients, and we have chosen to discuss this syndrome in Chapter 6.

## Multiple Sclerosis

A 19-year-old woman is seen in consultation for a severe depressive disorder, intermingled with histrionic features and emotional lability. On interview, she is distraught and complains of anorexia and sleep disturbance. An ambivalent relationship with a young man seems to be of dynamic importance. During the second session, she mentions that her left hand occasionally feels "numb."

---

*Clinical Rule 5.4:* In its infancy, the name given to insular sclerosis is hysteria.

---

### Discussion

Clinical rule 5.4 is not ours but was propounded by Dr. Buzzard in 1897. It remains a useful aphorism. There is evidence to suggest that patients with MS develop depressive affective disturbance with a greater frequency than do patients with other neurologic disorders, such as temporal lobe epilepsy and amyotrophic lateral sclerosis (Schiffer and Babigian, 1984). MS patients typically experience symptoms of their neurologic disease for 3–5 years before the

**Table 5.6**
Schumacher Criteria for Definite MS

| |
|---|
| Neurological examination reveals objective abnormalities of CNS function |
| Examination or history indicates involvement of two or more parts of CNS |
| CNS disease predominantly reflects white matter involvement |
| Involvement of CNS follows one or two patterns: |
| Two or more episodes, each lasting at least 24 hr and a month or more apart |
| Slow or stepwise progression of signs and symptoms over at least 6 months |
| Patient 10–50 years old at onset |
| Signs and symptoms cannot be better explained by other disease process |

diagnosis is made, and it is during this phase of the disease that they are most likely to be sent to psychiatry.

We do not have a laboratory test for MS, although magnetic resonance (MR) imaging may have a sensitivity in the range of 90%. The diagnosis still rests on the history and examination, indicating a relapsing/remitting white matter disease, usually with onset in early adult life. For many years the Schumacher diagnostic criteria applied (Schumacher *et al.*, 1965), and those criteria still convey the sense of the disease as one that is disseminated through CNS white matter in space and time (Table 5.6).

More recently, technologic advances in neurodiagnosis have been incorporated into the diagnostic criteria for MS (Poser *et al.*, 1983) (Table 5.7).

**Table 5.7**
New Diagnostic Criteria for Multiple Sclerosis (Poser Criteria)

| Category | Attacks | Clinical evidence | | Paraclinical evidence | CSF oligoclonal bands/IgG |
|---|---|---|---|---|---|
| Clinically definite MS | | | | | |
| 1 | 2 | 2 | | — | — |
| 2 | 2 | 1 | and | 1 | — |
| Laboratory-supported definite MS | | | | | |
| 1 | 2 | 1 | or | 1 | + |
| 2 | 1 | 2 | | — | + |
| 3 | 1 | 1 | and | 1 | + |
| Clinically probable MS | | | | | |
| 1 | 2 | 1 | | — | — |
| 2 | 1 | 2 | | — | — |
| 3 | 1 | 1 | and | 1 | — |
| Laboratory-supported probable | | | | | |
| 1 | 2 | — | | — | + |

Anatomic lesions identified by evoked responses, CT scan, or MR scan may now be used to identify second lesions in space.

## Demographics

There are two incidence peaks. Disease of the relapsing pattern tends to begin in early adult life and to be more common among women. Modal onset year for this disease type is approximately 26. The progressive form of disease tends to begin later in life, during the fourth and fifth decades. Men are more strongly represented in this group. The disease is more common among whites than blacks, and it is rare among Asians. The risk is higher by a factor of 3 or 4 for persons born and raised to the age of 14 in northern latitudes.

## Clinical History

Initial MS symptoms of optic neuritis or sensory changes commonly fail to come to medical attention. When the diagnosis is suspected, patients should be asked if there was ever a time earlier in life when one eye dimmed or went gray. Sensory abnormalities, which are usually described as numbness or tingling, should be sought. Unfortunately, MS-related symptoms may be exacerbated by stress and anxiety, so patients may tend to report them during periods of emotional turmoil. Unilateral or asymmetric sensory changes are of greater interest than symmetric ones. Urinary frequency is another common symptom, which some patients may fail to mention until asked. This particular symptom is not a common "functional" one.

## Psychotropic Drug Interactions

Tricyclic antidepressants may occasionally cause an MS patient to feel "weak all over," or "weak in the legs." All drugs with anticholinergic side effects may cause urinary retention in predisposed patients.

## Mental Status Examination

**Verbal Learning.** Cognitive deficits develop in a majority of MS patients, and they may be present early in the disease course (Ron, 1986). Verbal learning impairments in which spontaneous recall is dysfunctional but recognition recall normal are typical. Language and personality tend not to be affected.

**Depression.** The quality of the depressive episodes among MS patients is quite heterogeneous (Schiffer, 1987). Approximately two-thirds of these episodes are associated with progression or exacerbation of the neurologic disease, so new neurologic symptoms are present during the affective disturbance.

### General Medical Examination

Urinary retention. Bladder may be palpated, or postvoid residual volumes may exceed 100 ml.

### Neurologic Examination

Cranial Nerves. Abnormalities of optic discs and eye movements are especially common. Check for optic atrophy, or a pupil on one side that is sluggish or dilated compared with the other (Marcus-Gunn pupil). Nystagmus and disconjugate saccadic eye movements are common, especially of internuclear ophthalmoplegia pattern.

Motor. Weakness of upper motor neuron type and cerebellar ataxia are most common. Early midline cerebellar deficits may become evident only on testing tandem walking, or Romberg maneuvers.

Reflex. Check carefully for hyperreflexia or clonus. These findings are most useful when unilateral or asymmetric. Young women may demonstrate symmetric ankle clonus as a normal variation.

Sensory. Often abnormal; rarely reliable.

### Laboratory and Imaging

Brainstem auditory, visual, and somatosensory evoked responses are abnormal in a majority of MS patients, but sensitivity probably does not exceed 65% for any single test.

The CT scan occasionally shows an unexpected white matter lesion, but MR images are ten times as sensitive to areas of demyelination.

Lumbar puncture examination of CSF shows immunologic abnormalities in a majority of MS patients: oligoclonal banding of IgG which is not present in serum, and elevated CSF IgG compared with albumin or total protein (Rudick, 1985).

## Vasculopathy

The vasculitides include a family of diseases associated with inflammatory changes in the walls of blood vessels. They are classified on the basis of size and type of vessels involved, age of onset, and the nature of other systemic signs and laboratory changes that invariably accompany them. Most of these diseases produce an elevation of the erythrocyte sedimentation rate (ESR) at some time during their course. Most of them cause pain and systemic symptoms that are atypical for affective disorders.

There is one case report of a 46-year-old woman with periarteritis nodosa in whom the diagnosis of a depressive episode was entertained (Weddington *et al.*, 1986), but the depressive symptomatology occurred in the setting of an illness involving progressive cachexia, gastrointestinal pain, and myonecrosis. In giant cell arteritis (temporal arteritis), which almost universally affects people above the age of 55, a variety of depressivelike complaints may be seen (Russell, 1959). Once again, a majority of such patients have concomitant symptoms which are "red flags" for an affective diagnosis: headache, myalgias, diaphoresis, and jaw claudication.

*Migraine* is a noninflammatory disorder of arteriole and arterioles tone regulation, which may be associated with a sometimes mystifying array of systemic and neurologic symptoms. Sacks (1970) has reminded us that affective disturbances mimicking depression or anxiety may occur during the prodrome of a migraine attack. We agree that this is true, yet the context of these affective symptoms rarely causes serious diagnostic difficulty.

## MALIGNANCY, BRAIN TUMOR, AND DEPRESSION

### Discussion

In clinical terms, we will consider all mass lesions within the CNS as "tumors," since they cause symptoms by compressing brain tissue and by elevating intracerebral pressure. In this sense, a subdural hematoma acts like a tumor and demonstrates similar clinical clues during interview and examination. What is important for psychiatrists is to develop a clinical sense of when such mass lesions may be present. Malignant tumors that are outside the CNS may cause functional disturbance within the neuraxis by one of two mechanisms. *Metastasis* into the brain or spinal cord may occur, or remote effects may occur within the CNS from a distant tumor—so-called "paraneoplastic" effects. The mechanism(s) by which paraneoplastic syndromes occur are not well understood. Although paraneoplastic syndromes such as cerebellar degeneration must be more common than disturbances of mood and affect, it seems reasonable to maintain that paraneoplastic disorders of emotional states may occur.

Carcinoma of the pancreas is the extra-CNS malignancy that has been most often cited as capable of producing a paraneoplastic depressive disorder

(Perlas and Faillace, 1964; Fras *et al.*, 1967; Karliner, 1956). Fras and colleagues summarized the psychiatric literature as indicating a 10–20% frequency of depressive and anxiety symptoms early in the course of pancreatic carcinoma. In their interview series of 46 patients, 22 reported early depressive feelings or loss of ambition as the first symptoms of the disease. Only four of 64 colon carcinoma patients gave such a history. It should be noted that many of these patients have early vague or deep abdominal pain which is sometimes referred to the middorsal region. Middorsal pain, as opposed to cervical or lumbar pain, is uncommon as part of musculoskeletal strain or arthritis. More recently, a larger study has appeared comparing psychological profiles in patients with advanced pancreatic and gastric carcinomas (Holland *et al.*, 1986). In this study with more than 100 patients in each group, the authors found that the pancreatic cancer patients had higher self-ratings of depression, tension–anxiety, and total mood disturbance. One mechanism that might account for this association between pancreatic carcinoma and affective disturbance is the retroperitoneal location of some sympathetic catecholamine systems disrupted by the growing tumor.

Lishman (1978, p. 262) cites a frequency of one in 200 for undiagnosed primary or metastatic brain tumors among admissions to a psychiatric unit. A variety of clinical reports describe early depressive feelings among patients with expanding intracerebral masses (Burkle and Lipowski, 1978; Alarcon and Thweatt, 1983). When Remington and Rubert (1962) reviewed the presenting clinical condition among 30 brain tumor patients admitted to a state mental hospital, they found that the three most common signs or symptoms upon admission were depression, memory deficit, and combativeness. In another short, uncontrolled series of patients with hemispheric brain tumors who presented with behavioral symptoms, Donald and his colleagues (1972) reported a variety of atypical features. Their patients tended to complain of such symptoms as dizziness, headache, and memory loss in addition to affective disturbance. More clinical research needs to be done on such patients, but from the descriptions available, it seems that the "depression" that is described has often included psychomotor slowing as a prominent feature. Lethargy and impaired concentration are also described commonly, probably as a result of either prefrontal tumor location or early edema effects. We suspect that many of these patients would have demonstrated subtle or not-so-subtle abnormalities in other sections of the neurologic examination had they been examined carefully.

## Demographics

Pancreatic carcinoma is one of the malignancies of late middle age, with a mean age of onset in the 55- to 58-year range. It is neither a common nor a rare tumor, being found in 0.3–0.75% of large autopsy series. Sex ratios in pancreatic carcinoma "favor" men over women, with ratios reported in the range of 2:1. Smokers and patients with diabetes mellitus may be at greater risk.

Primary brain tumors are infrequent before the age of 10 and after the age of 70. The hemispheric tumors are generally diseases of early to middle adult life, without sexual predilection. Metastatic CNS tumors tend to occur in late middle life, when systemic primary cancer becomes more common. Breast and lung carcinomas together account for many such metastases. As in so many diseases, smokers are at much greater risk.

## Clinical History

Younger patients with primary brain tumors are the most difficult to sort out clinically. The lassitude, apathy, psychomotor slowing, and impaired concentration may be indistinguishable historically from an affective episode. In older patients one can be much more suspicious when such features occur for the first time. Headache is a difficult symptom to evaluate. Headaches associated with tumors are classically described as aching, continuous, worse after a period of recumbency, and associated with nausea. When such features are elicited spontaneously during open-ended questioning, they are worrisome. We have not generally found that direct questions concerning headache are of great diagnostic utility in many psychiatric patients. When a retroperitoneal malignancy is a possibility, one should listen for a history of nausea, vomiting, vague GI discomfort, and back pain. Constipation and diarrhea may occur. Weight loss has been reported universally with malignancies.

## Mental Status Examination

**Emotion.** The affective episodes that have been described have included progressive apathy and lassitude and, most importantly, GI pain. We feel compelled to invoke our somewhat histrionic clinical rule No. 5.5.

---

*Clinical Rule No. 5.5:* A first depressive episode after age 50 is cancer or other serious medical disease until proved otherwise.

---

**Concentration, Verbal and Visual Memory.** Impairments in these functions do not distinguish the mental status profiles of tumors from other affective episodes.

## General Medical Examination

Primary intracerebral tumors do not produce specific general medical findings. In carcinoma of the pancreas, the following findings should be sought: deep left or right upper-quadrant pain upon palpation; epigastric mass; jaundice; hepatomegaly; weight loss. Breast cancer patients are not so likely to present with cerebral metastasis as first clinical manifestation of their tumor. Heavy smokers with bronchogenic carcinoma, however, may present in this manner. Sometimes one can hear focal wheezes over the site of the tumor.

## Neurological Examination

The neurological examination is nonspecific in patients with pancreatic carcinoma but almost always demonstrates abnormalities in patients with symptomatic brain tumors.

Cranial Nerves. Papilledema and visual field loss or neglect are probably the most common signs.

Sensory. Tumors posterior to the central sulcus may produce sensory alteration only. The primary modalities (pain, temperature, vibration, proprioception) may be intact when cortical sensation (two-point discrimination; stereognosis; graphesthesia; topagnosia) shows impairment. The validity of sensory-only findings in a psychiatric patient is always limited.

Motor. Check for subtle signs of hemiparesis, such as pronator drift. During ambulation one has a good opportunity to observe early leg circumduction or decreased associated movements on one side.

Reflex. Check for abnormally brisk reflexes but especially for evidence of left/right asymmetry. Babinski signs are of great importance when the examiner has tumor in mind.

## Laboratory and Imaging

In pancreatic carcinoma 10–20% of patients have elevated amylase or lipase. Approximately the same number have fasting hyperglycemia or glycosuria. The glucose tolerance test is abnormal in 50%. Radiologically, an upper GI tract may show the tumor in advanced cases. Ultrasound and abdominal CT scans may show earlier lesions. A percutaneous transhepatic cholangiogram can visualize the biliary system.

For brain tumors the head CT scan remains the procedure of choice. Uncontrasted scans probably show more than 90% of tumors, depending on cell type, size, and location. The decision to perform a contrast scan in addition depends on the clinician's degree of suspicion that a tumor is present in the face of a normal uncontrasted scan.

## NEURODEGENERATIVE DISEASES AND DEPRESSION

### Idiopathic Parkinson's Disease

Over a period of months, a 55-year-old man gradually developed psychomotor slowing, loss of spontaneity, and flattening of emotional expression. He received the diagnosis of unipolar depressive disorder, and antidepressants were prescribed with modest benefit. On functional neurologic testing, he demonstrated one of the rigid abnormalities of muscle tone, masked facies, and disequilibrium during rapid turning in gait testing.

#### Discussion

Idiopathic Parkinson's disease is one of a family of degenerative diseases involving the basal ganglia and associated brainstem nuclei. Signs and symptoms vary somewhat among these various neurologic syndromes, but in idiopathic Parkinson's disease, prominent findings include masked facies, bradykinesia, difficulty initiating movements, ''lead pipe''-type increased muscle tone, resting tremor of ''pill-rolling'' type, postural instability and disequilibrium, and sometimes autonomic dysfunction.

Fortunately or unfortunately for psychiatrists, there is a subgroup of depressed patients whose signs and symptoms can mimic idiopathic Parkinson's disease, at least in part. Particularly, those depressive patients who have prominent psychomotor slowing may demonstrate bradykinesa, bradyphrenia, masked facies, small-step gait, and kyphotic posturing (Greden and Carroll, 1981; Sloman *et al.*, 1982). There are detailed case reports of patients with Parkinson's disease who received extensive psychiatric care until the disease had advanced sufficiently to make the diagnosis obvious (Kearney, 1964). We have seen such patients with some regularity at our hospital.

Neurologists face the converse of this clinical situation; depressive signs and symptoms are quite common among parkinsonian patients. Mayeux *et al.* (1984) have reviewed the clinical association between parkinsonism and depression and concluded that 40–50% of Parkinson's patients show signs of depression at any given time. The literature indicates that the depressive features, although common, are usually mild to moderate in severity. Suicide seems to be rare. The depression commonly develops at the time of clinical onset of the parkinsonism, and this probably accounts for the occasional diagnostic dilemma in psychiatry.

There are almost certainly neuroanatomic and neurophysiologic explanations for the clinical overlap between parkinsonism and depression. The rigid separation in our hospitals between diseases of mood and diseases of the motor system has little basis in neuroanatomy. Limbic system circuits and extrapyramidal circuits are quite intertwined both functionally and anatomically (Nauta, 1982), and there is evidence that Parkinson's disease may affect brainstem nuclei which provide some of the noradrenergic regulation of mood and affect (Javoy-Agid and Agid, 1980).

## Demographics

Idiopathic parkinsonism, as opposed to less common forms of parkinsonism secondary to toxins, infection, and stroke, is typically a disease of people over 50 years of age. One should be aware of the occasional youthful drug abuser who may develop parkinsonism as a consequence of attempted home laboratory synthesis of meperidine, which may produce MPTP (1-methyl,4-phenyl,1,2,3,6-tetrahydropyridine). In idiopathic Parkinson's disease, onset during the 40s occurs, but onset prior to age 40 is rare. The disease is shared equally by men and women, and familial clustering is uncommon. There does not seem to be a racial predilection.

### Clinical History

An early symptom of parkinsonism may be aching pains in the back or neck. Patients may complain of losing their balance more easily when a subway train accelerates. In young people for whom the disease is suspected, an encephalitislike episode should be sought in the history, or systemic drug abuse, which may have exposed them to MPTP.

## Psychotropic Drug Interaction

All dopamine-blocking drugs may cause parkinsonism.

Lithium has dopamine-blocking properties and may mimic certain parkinsonian features. Dysphagia may be more common than other signs. With the exception of the fine postural tremor, extrapyramidal signs due to lithium are usually a sign of advanced toxicity and are cause for immediate intervention.

Catecholamine-depleting drugs such as reserpine and tetrabenazine may cause parkinsonism.

## Mental Status Examination

Verbal Learning. Impairments of verbal learning and retention are common in moderately advanced parkinsonism.

Arousal and Language. Normal.

Higher Cognitive Processes. Some patients with parkinsonism develop impairments of abstract thinking and of concept formation, such as measured by the Wisconsin Card Sort test. They may also demonstrate difficulty in judging visual and postural vertical directions on tests that involve line orientation.

Thought Process. A slowing of the speed with which thought processes (bradyphrenia) may occur. This abnormality seems to improve with antiparkinsonian drug therapy to a greater extent than the other cognitive abnormalities.

## General Medical Examination

Skin. Seborrhea, especially facial, is common.

Autonomic. Postural hypotension and constipation are common. Hypertension itself tends to be uncommon among such patients.

## Neurological Examination

Cranial Nerves. Hypomimia; masked facies; up-gaze limitation.

Sensory. Normal.

Reflex. Normal.

Motor. Increased muscle tone of "lead pipe" quality; resting tremor which tends to be 3–5 cps in frequency. The tremor is exacerbated by focusing the patient's attention on the movement. Postural instability, especially when turning, may be seen, as well as kyphotic posturing and bradykinesia. The gait becomes small-step and festinating, and shows decreased associated movements.

## Laboratory and Imaging

There is no laboratory test for Parkinson's disease or for most other forms of parkinsonism, for that matter. The EEG shows nonfocal slowing in a majority of parkinsonian patients who are demented, and head CT may show nonspecific diffuse atrophy in such a population. These tests are more useful, however, in "ruling out" another disease than in "ruling in" parkinsonism, and they tend not to be helpful during the earliest phases of the disease, when diagnosis is most difficult.

## Alzheimer's Disease

After three consecutive psychiatric admissions for treatment of depression, a 60-year-old man has remained refractory to improvement. ECT conferred a modest lightening of his dysphoria during the first course but not after the second. Antidepressants and psychotherapies had been tried. Antidepressant toxicity limited the dosage of tricyclic antidepressants that could be given. After 6 months of such efforts, one interviewer noticed that the patient was beginning to make paraphasic errors.

### Discussion

Dr. Ewald ("Bud") Busse once remarked that he had observed a psychopathologic state occasionally in older patients that was undifferentiated or indeterminate between dementia and depression. Our clinical experience is consistent with this observation. We suspect that the most likely place to find such patients is among older persons with treatment-resistant depression. Dr. Busse speculated that this clinical state might be indeterminate in the sense that it could evolve in either direction toward clinical resolution or toward dementia, perhaps depending on treatment.

There is retrospective evidence that dementia of the Alzheimer's type may present as depressive illness. Liston (1977) reviewed the records of 50 patients with a diagnosis of "presenile dementia" and found that 75% of them had demonstrated depressive symptomatology early in their illness. Psychiatric diagnoses and treatments had been common. Reding *et al.* (1985) followed 28 depressed patients who had (erroneously?) been referred to their dementia clinic, and found that more than half of them developed frank dementia over a 3-year period. In retrospect, they felt that early clinical clues among those who would become demented were cognitive impairments, subtle abnormalities on neurologic examination, and confusion on low doses of antidepressants.

The problem, of course, is to distinguish early Alzheimer's dementia from an affective disorder with late onset. Despite impressive recent advances in neuroscientific investigations in Alzheimer's disease (see Kokmen, 1984, for a review), clinical judgment remains the mainstay of diagnosis. The NINCDS-ADRDA Work Group of the Department of Health and Human Services Task Force on Alzheimer's Disease has recently published criteria for the clinical diagnosis of Alzheimer's disease (McKhann *et al.*, 1984) (Table 5.8).

**Table 5.8**
Criteria for Clinical Diagnosis of Alzheimer's Disease

| |
|---|
| Probable Alzheimer's disease |
| Dementia, established by clinical examination and documented by formalized cognitive testing |
| Deficits in two or more areas of cognition |
| Progressive worsening of memory and other cognitive functions |
| No disturbance of consciousness |
| Onset between ages 40 and 90, most often after age 65 |
| Absence of systemic disorders or other brain diseases that in and of themselves could account for the progressive deficits in memory and cognition |
| Definitive Alzheimer's disease |
| Patient meets clinical criteria for probable Alzheimer's disease, and histopathologic evidence is present from biopsy or autopsy |

Unfortunately, depression itself is a disorder that can impair cognition as well as motor function (Wells, 1979). In the end, this diagnostic distinction becomes a matter of clinical judgment. In the suggestions that follow, we attempt to emphasize those features that have proved most useful in our clinical work.

## Demographics

Accurate prevalence and incidence studies for the dementias are not available, but a reasonable estimate is that 15–20% of persons above the age of 65 are demented (Terry and Davies, 1980). At least half of these people have dementia of the Alzheimer's type. There seems to be no sexual predilection for the disease, and it is probably equally common among whites and blacks. Familial clustering of the disease occurs, but not in every case (Nee *et al.*, 1983). There is continuing investigation into the question of whether Alzheimer's disease with onset prior to age 65 ("presenile dementia") is clinically or pathologically different from disease with onset after age 65 (Seltzer and Sherwin, 1983). Clinical features that may characterize the early-onset version of the disease include more prominent language disturbance, a shorter relative survival time, and a greater proportion of patients who are left-handed.

## Clinical History

In our history taking, when the diagnostic possibilities include early Alzheimer's disease versus affective disorder, we have found the clinical features listed in Table 5.9 useful to consider.

## Psychotropic Drug Interactions

We have the distinct clinical impression that Alzheimer's patients are exquisitely sensitive to drug side effects, often demonstrating acute confusional reactions or somnolence to relatively small doses. Such a response to a tricyclic antidepressant trial can be a warning about the diagnosis. Other drugs with anticholinergic properties and all types of dopaminergic medications may be especially likely to cause such disturbances.

## Mental Status Examination

**Verbal Learning.** Both depressed and Alzheimer's patients demonstrate deficits of verbal learning ability. As a matter of "style," the depressed patients tend to exaggerate less severe impairments demonstrated on mental status testing, and the Alzheimer's patients tend to minimize more severe deficits. Active or spontaneous recall of word lists may be severely impaired in both, but the depressed patients will often do surprisingly well on the test of recognition recall, which indicates that learning took place but that active retrieval has been impaired. The Alzheimer's patients typically have not learned many of the words at all.

**Language.** Depressed patients have normal language, but Alzheimer's patients may commonly demonstrate subtle signs of a fluent aphasia. Paraphasic

**Table 5.9**
Alzheimer's Disease Versus Late-Onset Affective Disorder

| Clinical features | Affective disorder | Alzheimer's disease |
|---|---|---|
| Date of onset for disorder | Onset reasonably discrete | Neither family nor patient can date onset—insidious beginning |
| Progression | Weeks to months | Months to years |
| Visuospatial difficulty: | | |
| Has the patient gotten lost? | No | Common |
| Memory disorder? | Family denies; patient insists | Patient denies; family insists |
| Psychomotor or gait change | Slows down | Speeds up or unchanged |
| Vocational performance change | Associates encourage patient to work; patient refuses | Associates encourage patient to leave work; patient refuses |
| Driving | Patient may cease driving of his own accord | Patient always continues to drive |

errors are common in their speech, and comprehension impairments with intact repetition may be present on formal testing (Kirshner, 1982). This pattern of aphasic errors is that of a "transcortical sensory" aphasia and is referrable to parietal and temporal neuropathologic changes which spare Wernicke's area itself. Differentiation from a Wernicke's aphasia, which is much more common in vascular disease, can be made by testing for the major functional impairments in repetition and reading of Wernicke's aphasia.

Visuospatial. Neuropathologically, Alzheimer's disease is not distributed uniformly through the hemispheres. Inferior parietal lobule involvement in the left hemisphere of right-handed patients produces a transcortical sensory aphasia. When the corresponding portion of the right hemisphere is involved, visuoconstructive skills are impaired. These patients get lost easily, especially in a novel environment. They have difficulty copying and recalling a geometric figure. They may have elements of anosognosia and denial of illness, also referrable to right-hemisphere involvement.

## General Medical Examination

No findings specifically suggestive of Alzheimer's disease. Indeed, we would hazard a clinical conjecture which we have found of some use in our work:

---

*Clinical Conjecture 5.1:* Any inpatient with more than three active medical problems does *not* have Alzheimer's disease.

---

Mathematical version of conjecture 5.1:

$$\frac{\text{Likelihood of Alzheimer's disease}}{\text{in a demented patient}} = \frac{1}{\text{No. of active medical problems}}$$

## Neurological Examination

Aside from the mental status abnormalities detailed earlier, the neurologic examination in early Alzheimer's dementia should be nonfocal. This is not to say that it should be normal. A number of "release signs" or disinhibitory phenomena may appear as this degenerative disease progresses. In Jenkyn's controlled study, he found that the following release signs *each* had a false-negative rate less than 60% in distinguishing demented patients from normal controls (Jenkyn, 1977) (Table 5.10).

In this study, Jenkyn also found that when three or more release signs were present, the likelihood of a "false-positive" diagnosis of diffuse cerebral dysfunction fell to 11% or less. Still, we recommend caution in using these

**Table 5.10**
Release Signs with False-Negative Rates Less Than 60%

| |
|---|
| Nuchocephalic response |
| Glabellar tap |
| Suck reponse |
| Up-gaze restriction |
| Down-gaze restriction |
| Saccadic pursuits |
| Lateral gaze impersistence |
| Paratonia |

release signs in the diagnosis of dementia. In our view there has been insufficient standardization of such tests in current clinical research, and there is insufficient information available concerning the ''natural'' appearance of these signs during the course of normal aging. We prefer to use them as suggestive or confirmatory findings, in a manner similar to the way in which we use the laboratory testing discussed later. In a sense, they become highly individualized portions of the neurologic examination, of more use to clinicians who have developed familiarity with them.

### Laboratory and Imaging

CT scans, MR scans, and EEGs cannot be used to diagnose Alzheimer's dementia. There is a general correlation between increasing ventricular and sulcal size by CT scan and clinical dementia, but in any given case the scan may be normal (Damasio *et al.*, 1983; Albert *et al.*, 1984). Generalized slowing of the background frequency by EEG also helps to distinguish demented from normals when large groups are examined (Weiner and Schuster, 1956; Roberts *et al.*, 1978), but it is typically not helpful for a given individual. We consider these imaging tests more useful in *ruling out* another cause of dementia such as stroke or tumor than in *ruling in* Alzheimer's disease. There are no laboratory tests available that confirm the presence of Alzheimer's disease.

## INFECTION

### Discussion

In our experience, meningitis and encephalitis do not commonly mimic affective disorders. People with bacterial, viral, fungal, and protozoal infections of the CNS *look* sick and *feel* sick. They are usually febrile and delirious. Triage nurses rarely send such patients to psychiatry. The nonbacterial opportunists are more likely to produce an indolent clinical course, with behavioral and affective change. In older days, neurosyphilis was by far the most common organism in such a clinical setting. Today, these opportunist infections are more likely to occur in the setting of chronic, debilitating medical illness, especially one whose treatment has compromised immune-system function. The behavioral syndromes associated with human immune deficiency virus (HIV) infections must be considered among high-risk populations, and chronic Epstein-Barr virus infection among young people is a serious consideration.

Infections associated with the HIV were first recognized in the United States in 1981. The causative virus is one of several human T-lymphotropic retroviruses, which have the following features: (1) tropism for $OKT_4^+$ lymphocytes; (2) presence of reverse transcriptose of high molecular weight; (3) capacity to inhibit T-cell function or to kill T cells. For recent reviews of the immunology of this virus and of the variety of clinical phenomena that may be seen in the acquired immune deficiency syndrome (AIDS) it produces, see Levy *et al.* (1985) and Navia and Price (1987).

Groups of patients who seem to be at risk for AIDS include: (1) homosexual or bisexual males; (2) intravenous drug users; (3) heterosexual partners of groups (1) and (2); (4) patients who require multiple blood transfusions; and (5) children of high-risk parents.

It seems clear that a substantial number of persons suffering from AIDS (perhaps the majority) will develop the AIDS dementia complex, a syndrome characterized generally by progressive cognitive loss, spasticity, and weakness. During the early phases of this syndrome, behavioral signs and symptoms may predominate (Rundell *et al.*, 1986). Prominent apathy, anergy, and social withdrawal are common findings and may be mistaken for signs of a depressive disorder (Hollander and Levy, 1987). Psychosis has been described as well, but it has been our experience that the syndrome more often looks like an affective disorder.

Another infection–affective disorders link under investigation includes the association of chronic Epstein-Barr virus infection with a syndrome of lassitude and dysphoria (Delisi *et al.*, 1986; Amsterdam *et al.*, 1986). There is a controversy concerning how widespread such an association might be. It seems reasonable to suspect an underlying EBV infection when depressive symptomatology is accompanied by lymphadenopathy, hyperpyrexia, fever, or hepatitis. As in all of the syndromes discussed in this book, when one embarks upon laboratory testing unguided by clinical clues, time and money are wasted.

Despite the reputation for grandiose and expansive behavior by neurosyphilis patients, a depressivelike clinical picture early in the disease appears to be much more common. When Dewhurst (1969) reviewed 91 neurosyphilis patients admitted to mental hospitals during the antibiotic era, he found that the commonest early symptoms of the disease included depression, headache, forgetfulness, insomnia, irritability, apathy, and epilepsy. Interestingly, 30.8% of this group had initially received psychiatric diagnoses of reactive, endogenous, involutional, and senile depression. A small percentage (14.3%) had received diagnoses of dementia. Most of these patients were midlife by the time of their psychiatric diagnoses, reinforcing our clinical rule No. 5.5.

## Demographics

The high-risk groups for AIDS are listed in the preceding section. Neurosyphilis affects men more commonly than women, with a ratio of approximately 3:1. It is *not* a young person's disease, but has a modal onset age in the late 40s or early 50s. Most of the Epstein-Barr patients have been adults in the third or fourth decade, without sexual predilection.

## Clinical History

History taking for sexually transmitted diseases requires some tact. Many people are reticent in discussing their sexual adjustment and behaviors with physicians, and perhaps more so with mental health clinicians. For the AIDS syndrome one can ask about unusual infections: candidiasis of mouth or esophagus, atypical pneumonia such as pneumocystis, or particularly severe herpes ulcerations. If the suspicion of AIDS occurs to the clinician, direct questions concerning sexual adjustment and contacts must be asked. For neurosyphilis we have found useful clues at times from questions such as the following: Previous treatment with penicillin? Skin rash? Rejection from army? Denial of marriage license? Contact with people who had the clap?

## Mental Status Examination

### In AIDS Dementia

*Thought process.* Typically slowed, with particular difficulty in tasks involving rapid alternation of psychological set. They may often complain of difficulty following themes on television programs or in books.

*Verbal memory.* Impaired, including both active and recognition recall.

*Language.* Typically normal, except for decreased fluency as the disease progresses.

### In Neurosyphilis

*Verbal memory.* Impaired early, but pattern will depend on the neuroanatomy involved in the particular individual.

*Aphasia, agnosia, apraxia.* Abnormalities in one or more of these functions are typical in this essentially cortical dementia. No precise pattern can be described.

## General Medical Examination

Nonspecific in neurosyphilis. In AIDS, one may see evidence of mucosal candida, herpes, or Kaposi's sarcoma in skin. In EBV suspects, check for pharyngitis, enlarged lymph nodes, or hepatomegaly.

## Neurological Examination

### Neurosyphilis

*Cranial nerves.* Optic atrophy; pupillary abnormalities—Argyll Robertson pupils are small and irregular and react to accommodation but not to light. *Any* abnormality of pupillary size, shape, or reactivity may be seen, however. Dysarthia was a frequent sign.

*Motor.* Postural tremor of outstretched hands; gait abnormalities are common when posterior columns of spinal cord are affected; wide-based, "foot-slapping" patterns.

*Sensory.* Any pattern of impairment may be seen, but posterior column modalities (vibration and proprioception) may be selectively involved.

*Reflex.* Upper motor neuron pattern hyperreflexia with Babinski signs and asymmetry left/right are most common.

AIDS. In AIDS dementia complex, accompanying neurologic signs often include gait ataxia, diffuse hyperreflexia, and leg spasticity. Babinski signs may be present. Peripheral neuropathic sensory findings are common and are usually associated with CNS viral infection as well as peripheral involvement.

## Laboratory and Imaging

The most reliable tests for AIDS include (1) ELISA assay for HIV antibody in serum or CSF; (2) viral cultures, in centers where available; and (3) T-cell subsets. In AIDS patients there is a reversal of the ratio in peripheral blood of the two major T-cell subsets. These subpopulations are identified by antigens Leu 3/$OKT_4$ (T helper) and Leu 2/$OKT_8$ (T suppressor/cytotoxic). Normal percentages are 64%/36%, respectively, of total T cells. A normal ratio is approximately 1.7, and a reversed ratio would be approximately 0.5.

It is surprising how much clinical judgment must be brought to bear in deciding the evaluation for possible neurosyphilis (Table 5.11), as well as the treatment. The diagnostic issue is made the more difficult since the antibiotic

**Table 5.11**
Laboratory Tests for Neurosyphilis

| Test | Specificity | Comment |
|---|---|---|
| Serum VDRL | 50% false negatives | False positives common, due to normal aging, autoimmune disease. Partial treatment may normalize serum VDRL |
| Serum FTA-ABS (fluorescent typonemal antibody absorption) | 95% sensitive to syphilis infection | Does *not* prove neurosyphilis |
| Serum MHA-TP (treponema micro-hemagglutination assay) | 95% sensitive to syphilis infection | Does *not* prove neurosyphilis |
| CSF VDRL | Almost diagnostic for neurosyphilis. False negatives 30–40% | May be positive when serum VDRL is negative |
| CSF increased total protein (<50 mg/dl) | Present in 60% of neurosyphilis cases | May be a sign of disease activity |
| CSF pleocytosis (<7 WBC/ml) | Present in 50–60% of neurosyphilis cases | Cells are usually lymphocytes, and count is often low (8–10 WBC/$\mu$l). A good sign of disease activity |

protocol for neurosyphilis is considerably more ambitious than for primary or secondary syphilis. Our general recommendation is that lumbar puncture should be performed for anyone with a positive serum FTA-ABS and *any* mental status or neurological abnormality. If the CSF VDRL is positive, the treatment regimen should be administered. If pleocytosis or elevated protein is present in CSF, clinical judgment must be exercised, but our bias remains in favor of treatment.

## EPILEPSY AND DEPRESSION

Depression may be the most common psychopathological condition found among patients with epilepsy (Trimble, 1985), but epileptics are not often confused with depressed patients. We have not yet participated in a clinical case seminar in which the differential diagnosis wavered between epilepsy and depression. This, of course, is quite different from the situation regarding partial complex epilepsy and paranoid psychotic states. The reader is referred to Chapter 8 for discussion of this diagnostic problem.

## STROKE AND VASCULAR DISEASE

Again, there is very interesting literature concerning an association between left frontal lobe stroke and depression (Robinson *et al.*, 1985, 1986), but the neurology of these patients tends to be anything but subtle. These patients are teaching us something about hemispheric lateralization and affective disorders, but they do not try our psychodiagnostic acumen.

## TRAUMA

There are scattered reports of individuals who developed depressive or bipolar affective disorders after head trauma (Parker, 1957). However, the trauma seems to have been of considerable severity, and the posttraumatic condition is accompanied by considerable cognitive damage. For these reasons, we will not discuss such syndromes further.

## REFERENCES

Alarcon, R. D., and Thweatt, R. W. A case of subdural hematoma mimicking severe depression with conversion-like symptoms. *Am. J. Psychiatry*, 1983, **140,** 1360–1361.

Albert, M., Naeser, M. A., Levine, H. L., and Garvey, A. J. Ventricular size in patients with presenile dementia of the Alzheimer's type. *Arch. Neurol.*, 1984, **41,** 1258–1263.

Anand, B. K., and Dua, S. Stimulation of limbic system of brain in waking animals. *Science*, 1955, **122,** 1139.

Amsterdam, J. D., Henle, W., Winokur, A., Wolkowitz, O. M., Pickar, D., and Paul, S. M. Serum antibodies to Epstein-Barr virus in patients with major depressive disorder. *Am. J. Psychiatry*, 1986, **143,** 1592–1596.

Aron, D. C., Tyrrell, J. B., Fitzgerald, P. A., Findling, J. W., and Forsham, P. H. Cushing's syndrome: Problems in diagnosis. *Medicine*, 1981, **60,** 25–35.

Beresford, T. P., Hall, R. C. W., Wilson, F. C., and Blow, F. Clinical laboratory data in psychiatric outpatients. *Psychosomatics*, 1985, **26,** 731–744.

Bonnyns, M., Van Haelst, L., and Bastenie, P. A. Asymptomatic atrophic thyroiditis. *Horm. Res.*, 1982, **16,** 338–344.

Borer, M. S., and Bhanot, V. K. Hyperparathyroidism: Neuropsychiatric manifestations. *Psychosomatics*, 1985, **26,** 597–601.

Burkle, F. M., and Lipowski, Z. J. Colloid cyst of the third ventricle presenting as a psychiatric disorder. *Am. J. Psychiatry*, 1978, **135,** 373–374.

Buzzard, T. *Lancet*, 1897, No. 3827, 1–4.

Caine, E. D., and Polinsky, R. J. Haloperidol-induced dysphoria in patients with Tourette syndrome. *Am. J. Psychiatry*, 1979, **136,** 1216–1217.

Calabrese, J. R., Gulledge, A. D., Hahn, K., Skwerer, R., Kotz, M., Schumaker, O. P., Gupta, M. K., Krupp, N., and Gold, P. W. Autoimmune thyroiditis in manic-depressive patients treated with lithium. *Am. J. Psychiatry*, 1985, **142,** 1318–1321.

Carpenter, P. C. Cushing's syndrome: Update of diagnosis and management. *Clin. Pract.*, 1986, **61,** 49–58.

Casper, R. C., Redmond, D. E., Katz, M. M., Schaffer, C. B., Davis, J. M., and Koslow, S. H. Somatic symptoms in primary affective disorder. *Arch. Gen. Psychiatry*, 1985, **42**, 1098–1104.

Cohen, K. L., and Swigar, M. E. Thyroid function screening in psychiatric patients. *JAMA*, 1979, **242**, 254–257.

Damasio, H., Eslinger, P., Damasio, A. R., Rizzo, M., Huang, H. K., and Demeter, S. Quantitative computed tomographic analysis in the diagnosis of dementia. *Arch. Neurol.*, 1983, **40**, 715–719.

Delisi, L. E., Nurnberger, J. I., Simmons-Alling, S., and Gershon, E. S. Epstein-Barr virus and depression. *Arch. Gen. Psychiatry*, 1986, **43**, 815–816.

Dewhurst, K. The neurosyphilitic psychoses today: A survey of 91 cases. *Br. J. Psychiatry*, 1969, **115**, 31–38.

*Diagnostic and Statistical Manual of Mental Disorders*, 3d ed., rev. Washington, D.C.: American Psychiatric Association, 1987.

Donald, A. G., Still,, C. N., and Pearson, J. M. Behavioral symptoms with intracranial neoplasm. *South. Med. J.*, 1972, **65**, 1006–1009.

Dowling, R. H., and Knox, S. J. Somatic symptoms in depressive illness. *Br. J. Psychiatry*, 1964, **110**, 720–722.

Editorial. Now read this: The SI units are here. *JAMA*, 1986, **255**, 2329–2339.

Feighner, J. P., Robins, E., Guze, S. B., Woodruff, R. A., Winokur, G., and Munoz, R. Diagnostic criteria for use in psychiatric research. *Arch. Gen. Psychiatry*, 1972, **26**, 57–63.

Fras, I., Litin, E. M., and Pearson, J. S. Comparison of psychiatric symptoms in carcinoma of the pancreas with those in some other intra-abdominal neoplasms. *Am. J. Psychiatry*, 1967, **123**, 1553–1562.

Gatewood, J. W., Organ, C. H., and Mead, B. T. Mental changes associated with hyperparathyroidism. *Am. J. Psychiatry*, 1975, **132**, 129–132.

Gloor, P., Andre, O., Quesney, L. F., Andermann, F., and Horowitz, S. The role of the limbic system in experiential phenomena of temporal lobe epilepsy. *Ann. Neurol.*, 1982, **12**, 129–144.

Gold, M. S., Pottash, A. L. C., and Extein, I. Hypothyroidism and depression. *JAMA*, 1981a, **245**, 1919–1922.

Gold, M. S., Pottash, A. L. C., Mueller, E. A., and Extein, I. Grades of thyroid failure in 100 depressed and anergic psychiatric patients. *Am. J. Psychiatry*, 1981b, **138**, 253–255.

Gold, M. S., Pottash, A. L. C., and Extein, I. "Symptomless" autoimmune thyroiditis in depression. *Psychiatry Res.*, 1982, **6**, 261–269.

Gold, P. W., Loriaux, D. L., Roy, A., Kling, M. A., Calabrese, J. R., Kellner, C. H., Nieman, L. K., Post, R. M., Pickar, D., Gallucci, W., Augerinos, P., Paul, S., Oldfield, E. H., Cutler, G. B., and Chrousos, G. P. Responses to corticotropin-releasing hormone in the hypercortisolism of depression and Cushing's disease. *N. Engl. J. Med.*, 1986, **314**, 1329–1335.

Goodwin, F. K., and Bunney, W. E. Depression following reserpine: A reevaluation. *Semin. Psychiatry*, 1971, **3**, 435–448.

Goodwin, F. K., Murphy, D. L., Brodie, H. K. H., and Bunney, W. E. L-Dopa, catecholamines, and behavior: A clinical and biochemical study in depressed patients. *Biol. Psychiatry*, 1970, **2**, 341–366.

Greden, J. F., and Carroll, B. J. Psychomotor function in affective disorders: An overview of new monitoring techniques. *Am. J. Psychiatry*, 1981, **138**, 1441–1448.

Hall, R. C. W. Depression. In Hall, R. C. W. (ed.): *Psychiatric Presentations of Medical Illness: Somatopsychic Disorders*. New York: SP Medical and Scientific Books, 1980.

Holland, J. C., Korzun, A. H., Tross, S., Silberfarb, P., Perry, M., Comis, R., and Oster, M. Comparative psychological disturbance in patients with pancreatic and gastric cancer. *Am. J. Psychiatry*, 1986, **143**, 982–986.

Hollander, H., and Levy, J. A. Neurologic abnormalities and recovery of human immunodeficiency virus from cerebrospinal fluid. *Ann. Intern. Med.*, 1987, **106,** 692–695.

Hudson, J. I., Hudson, M. S., Griffing, G. T., Melby, J. C., and Pope, H. G. Phenomenology and family history of affective disorder in Cushing's Disease. *Am. J. Psych.*, 1987, **144,** 951–953.

Javoy-Agid, F., and Agid, Y. Is the mesocortical dopaminergic system involved in Parkinson's disease? *Neurology (NY),* 1980, **30,** 1326–1330.

Jenkyn, L. R. Clinical signs in diffuse cerebral dysfunction. *J. Neurol. Neurosurg. Psychiatry,* 1977, **40,** 956–966.

Karliner, W. Psychiatric manifestations of cancer of the pancreas. *N.Y. State J. Med.*, 1956, **56,** 2251–2252.

Karpati, G., and Frame, B. Neuropsychiatric disorders in primary hyperparathyroidism: Clinical analysis with review of the literature. *Arch. Neurol.*, 1964, **10,** 387–397.

Kearney, T. R. Parkinson's disease presenting as depressive illness. *J. Irish Med. Assoc.*, 1964, **54,** 117–119.

Kelly, W. F., Checkley, S. A., Bender, D. A., and Mashiter, K. Cushing's syndrome and depression: A prospective study of 26 patients. *Br. J. Psychiatry,* 1983, **142,** 16–19.

Kirshner, H. S. Language disorders in dementia. In Kirshner, H. S., and Freemon, F. R. (eds.): *The Neurology of Aphasia,* Chap. 11. Lisse, The Netherlands: Swets and Zeitlinger B. V., 1982.

Kokmen, E. Dementia-Alzheimer type. *Mayo Clin. Proc.*, 1984, **59,** 35–42.

Lake, C. R., and Ziegler, M. G. (eds.). *The Catecholamines in Psychiatric and Neurologic Disorders.* London: Butterworth, 1985.

Levy, R. M., Bredesen, D. E., and Rosenblum, M. L. Neurological manifestations of the acquired immunodeficiency syndrome (AIDS): Experience at UCSF and review of the literature. *J. Neurosurg.*, 1985, **62,** 475–495.

Lishman, W. A. *Organic Psychiatry: The Psychological Consequences of Cerebral Disorder.* Oxford, U.K.: Blackwell, 1978.

Liston, E. H. Occult presenile dementia. *J. Nerv. Ment. Dis.*, 1977, **164,** 263–267.

Loosen, P. T., and Prange, A. J. Serum thyrotropin response to thyrotopin-releasing hormone in psychiatric patients: A review. *Am. J. Psychiatry,* 1982, **139,** 405–416.

Loosen, P. T., and Prange, A. J. Hormones of the thyroid axis and behavior. In Nemeroff, C. B., and Dunn, A. J. (eds.): *Peptides, Hormones, and Behavior.* New York: Spectrum, 1984, pp. 533–577.

Mann, J. J., Brown, R. P., Halper, J. P., Sweeney, J. A., Kocsis, J. H., Stokes, P. E., and Bilezikian, J. P. Reduced sensitivity of lymphocyte beta-adrenergic receptors in patients with endogenous depression and psychomotor agitation. *N. Engl. J. Med.*, 1985, **313,** 715–720.

Mayeux, R., Williams, J. B. W., Stern, Y., and Cote, L. Depression and Parkinson's disease. *Adv. Neurol.*, 1984, **40,** 241–250.

McKhann, G., Drachman, D., Folstein, F., Katzman, R., Price, D., and Stadlan, E. M. Clinical diagnosis of Alzheimer's disease: Report of the NINCDS-ADRDA work group under the auspices of department of health and human services task force on Alzheimer's disease. *Neurology* (NY), 1984, **34,** 939–944.

*Mental Disorders: Glossary and Guide to Their Classification in Accordance with the Ninth Revision of the International Classification of Diseases.* Geneva: World Health Organization, 1978.

Michael, R. P., and Gibbons, J. L. Interrelationships between the endocrine system and neuropsychiatry. *Int. Rev. Neurobiol.*, 1963, **5,** 243–302.

National Diabetes Data Group. Classification and diagnosis of diabetes mellitus and other categories of glucose intolerance. *Diabetes,* 1979, **28,** 1039–1057.

Nauta, W. J. H. Limbic innervation of the striatum. In Friedhoff, A. J., and Chase, T. N. (eds.): *Gilles de la Tourette Syndrome*. New York: Raven Press, 1982, pp. 41–47.

Navia, B. A., and Price, R. W. The acquired immunodeficiency syndrome dementia complex as the presenting or sole manifestation of human immunodeficiency virus infection. *Arch. Neurol.*, 1987, **44,** 65–69.

Nee, L. E., Polinsky, R. J., Eldridge, R., Weingartner, H., Smallberg, S., and Ebert, M. A family with histologically confirmed Alzheimer's disease. *Arch. Neurol.*, 1983, **40,** 203–208.

Parker, N. Manic depressive psychosis following head injury. *Med. J. Aust.*, 1957, **2,** 20–22.

Perlas, A. P., and Faillace, L. A. Psychiatric manifestations of carcinoma of the pancreas. *Am. J. Psychiatry,* 1964, **121,** 182.

Petersen, P. Psychiatric disorders in primary hyperparathyroidism. *J. Clin. Endocrinol. Metab.*, 1968, **28,** 1491–1495.

Poser, C. M., Paty, D. W., Scheinberg, L., McDonald, W. I., Davis, F. A., Ebers, G. C., Johnson, K. P., Sibley, W. A., Silberberg, D. H., and Tourtellotte, W. W. New diagnostic criteria for multiple sclerosis: Guidelines for research protocols. *Ann. Neurol.*, 1983, **13,** 227–231.

Post, R. M., and Ballenger, J. C. (eds.). *Neurobiology of Mood Disorders*. Baltimore: Williams and Wilkins, 1984.

Pritchard, B. N. C., Johnston, A. W., Hill, I. D., and Rosenheim, M. L. Bethanidine, guanethidine, and methyldopa in the treatment of hypertension: A within-patient comparison. *Br. Med. J.*, 1968, **I,** 135–144.

Quetsch, R. M., Achor, R. W. P., Litin, E. M., and Faucett, R. L. Depressive reaction in hypertensive patients: A comparison of those treated with rauwolfia and those receiving no specific antihypertensive treatment. *Circulation,* 1959, **19,** 366–375.

Reding, M., Haycox, J., and Blass, J. Depression in patients referred to a dementia clinic. *Arch. Neurol.*, 1985, **42,** 894–896.

Remington, F. B., and Rubert, S. L. Why patients with brain tumors come to a psychiatric hospital: A thirty year survey. *Am. J. Psychiatry,* 1962, **119,** 256–257.

Roberts, M. A., McGeorge, A. P., and Caird, F. I. Electroencephalography and computerized tomography in vascular and non-vascular dementia in old age. *J. Neurol. Neurosurg. Psychiatry,* 1978, **41,** 903–906.

Robinson, R. G., Lipsey, J. R., and Price, T. R. Diagnosis and clinical management of post-stroke depression. *Psychosomatics,* 1985, **26,** 769–778.

Robinson, R. G., Lipsey, J. R., Rao, K., and Price, T. R. Two year longitudinal study of post stroke mood disorders: Comparison of acute-onset with delayed-onset depression. *Am. J. Psychiatry,* 1986, **143,** 1238–1244.

Rodin, G., and Voshart, K. Depression in the medically ill: An overview. *Am. J. Psychiatry,* 1986, **143,** 696–705.

Ron, M. A. Multiple sclerosis: Psychiatric and psychometric abnormalities. *J. Psychosom. Res.*, 1986, **30,** 3–11.

Rudick, R. A. Humoral immunity in multiple sclerosis clinical and investigative aspects. *Semin. Neurol.*, 1985, **5,** 107–116.

Rundell, J. R., Wise, M. G., and Ursano, R. J. Three cases of AIDS-related psychiatric disorders. *Am. J. Psychiatry,* 1986, **143,** 777–778.

Russell, R. W. R. Giant cell arteritis: A review of 35 cases. *Q. J. Med.*, 1959, **28,** 471–489.

Sacks, O. W. *Migraine: The Evolution of a Common Disorder*. London: Faber, 1970.

Schiffer, R. B. The spectrum of depression in multiple sclerosis: An approach for clinical management. *Arch. Neurol.*, 1987, **44,** 596–599.

Schiffer, R. B., and Babigian, H. M. Behavioral disorders in multiple sclerosis, temporal lobe epilepsy, and amyotrophic lateral sclerosis. *Arch. Neurol.*, 1984, **41,** 1067–1069.

Schumacher, G. A., Beebe, G., Kibler, R. E., Kurland, L. T., Kurzke, J. F., McDowell, F., Nagler, B., Sibley, W. A., Tourtellotte, W. W., and Willmon, T. L. Problems of experimental trials of therapy in multiple sclerosis: Report by the panel on the evaluation of experimental trials of therapy in multiple sclerosis. *Ann. N.Y. Acad. Sci.*, 1965, **122,** 552–568.

Seltzer, B., and Sherwin, I. A comparison of clinical features in early- and late-onset primary degenerative dementia: One entity or two? *Arch. Neurol.*, 1983, **40,** 143–146.

Shader, R. I. *Psychiatric Complications of Medical Drugs*. New York: Raven Press, 1972.

Sloman, L., Berridge, M., Homatidis, M. A., Hunter, D., and Duck, T. Gait patterns of depressed patients and normal subjects. *Am. J. Psychiatry,* 1982, **139,** 94–97.

Smigan, L., Wahlin, A., Jacobsson, L., and Von Knorring, L. Lithium therapy and thyroid function tests: A prospective study. *Neuropsychobiology,* 1984, **11,** 39–43.

Spiger, M., Jubiz, W., Meikle, A. W., West, C. D., and Tylor, F. H. Single-dose metyrapone test: Review of a four-year experience. *Arch. Intern. Med.*, 1975, **135,** 698–700.

Starkman, M. N., Schteingart, D. E., and Schork, M. A. Correlation of bedside cognitive and neuropsychological tests in patients with Cushing's syndrome. *Psychosomatics,* 1986, **27,** 508–511.

Taylor, J. W. Depression in thyrotoxicosis. *Am. J. Psychol.*, 1975, **132,** 552–553.

Terry, R. D., and Davies, P. Dementia of the Alzheimer type. *Annu. Rev. Neurosci.*, 1980, **3,** 77–95.

Thomas, F. B., Mazzaferri, E. L., and Skillman, T. G. Apathetic thyrotoxicosis: A distinctive clinical and laboratory entity. *Ann. Intern. Med.*, 1970, **72,** 679–685.

Trethowan, W. H., and Cobb, S. Neuropsychiatric aspects of Cushing's syndrome. *Arch. Neurol. Psychiatry,* 1952, **67,** 283–309.

Trimble, M. R. Psychiatric and psychological aspects of epilepsy. In Morseli, P. L., Porter, R. J. (eds.): *Interictal Psychoses of Epilepsy,* Chap. 16. London: Butterworth, 1984.

Varadaraj, R., and Cooper, A. J. Addison's disease presenting with psychiatric symptoms. *Am. J. Psychiatry,* 1986, **143,** 553–554 (letter).

Waal, H. J. Propranolol induced depression. *Br. Med. J.*, 1967, **2,** 50 (letter).

Warnes, H. Physical illness in the psychiatric patient. In Koranyi, E. K. (ed.): *Physical Illness in the Psychiatric Patient.* Springfield, IL: Charles C. Thomas, 1982, pp. 119–137.

Weddington, W. W., Cook, E. H., and Denson, M. W. Periarteritis nodosa mimicking an affective disorder. *Psychosomatics,* 1986, **27,** 449–451.

Weiner, H., and Schuster, D. B. The electroencephalogram in dementia: Some preliminary observations and correlations. *Electroencephalography,* 1956, **8,** 479–488.

Wells, C. E. Pseuododementia. *Am. J. Psychiatry,* 1979, **136,** 895–900.

Whelan, T. B., Schteingart, D. E., Starkman, M. N., and Smith, A. Neuropsychological deficits in Cushing's syndrome. *J. Nerv. Ment. Dis.*, 1980, **168,** 753–757.

Whybrow, P. C., and Horwitz, T. Psychological disturbances associated with endocrine disease and hormone therapy. In Sachar, E. J. (ed.): *Hormones, Behavior, and Psychopathology.* New York: Raven Press, 1976, pp. 125–143.

Whybrow, P. C., Prange, A. J., and Treadway, C. R. Mental changes accompanying thyroid gland dysfunction. *Arch. Gen. Psychiatry,* 1969, **20,** 48–63.

Williams, D. The structure of emotions reflected in epileptic experiences. *Brain,* 1956, **79,** 29–67.

Zimmerman, M., Coryell, W., and Pfohl, B. The validity of the dexamethasone suppression test as a marker for endogenous depression. *Arch. Gen. Psychiatry,* 1986, **43,** 347–355.

# 6

# Manic Syndrome

## DSM-III-R Diagnosis

*Manic Episode*

A. A distinct period of abnormally and persistently elevated, expansive, or irritable mood.

B. During the period of mood disturbance, at least three of the following symptoms have persisted (four if the mood is only irritable) and have been present to a significant degree:
   1. inflated self-esteem or grandiosity
   2. decreased need for sleep, e.g., feels rested after only 3 hr of sleep
   3. more talkative than usual or pressure to keep talking
   4. flight of ideas or subjective experience that thoughts are racing
   5. distractibility, i.e., attention too easily drawn to unimportant or irrelevant external stimuli
   6. increase in goal-directed activity (either socially, at work or school, or sexually) or psychomotor agitation
   7. excessive involvement in pleasurable activities which have a high potential for painful consequences, e.g., the person engages in unrestrained buying sprees, sexual indiscretions, or foolish business investments

C. Mood disturbance sufficiently severe to cause marked impairment in occupational functioning or in usual social activities or relationships with others, or to necessitate hospitalization to prevent harm to self or others.

D. At no time during the disturbance have there been delusions or hallucinations for as long as 2 weeks in the absence of prominent mood symptoms (i.e., before the mood symptoms developed or after they have remitted).

## ICD-9 Diagnosis

*Manic-Depressive Psychosis, Manic Type.* Mental disorders characterized by states of elation or excitement out of keeping with the patient's circumstances and varying from enhanced liveliness (hypomania) to violent, almost uncontrollable excitement, aggression, and anger, flight of ideas, distractibility, impaired judgment, and grandiose ideas are common.

Krauthammer and Klerman (1978) have made the point that "manic episode" refers to a syndrome with many etiologies, not to a diagnosis in itself. Such an approach commends itself for each of the major mental status syndromes discussed in this book. In the case of secondary mania,* the plethora of medical and neurologic conditions in which the syndrome has been described makes one dubious that any single pathophysiology could be at work (see Table 6.1). As in the other chapters of this book, we have italicized those etiologies we have judged common enough to be discussed in the text.

Our usual caveat applies to Table 6.1: it is too long to be carried in one's head, and too hard to find if in one's pocket. Moreover, secondary manic episodes that occur during the course of medical or neurologic disease are not nearly so common as the secondary depressive syndromes. And despite the diversity of etiologies in Table 6.1, it has been our experience that only a few of these syndromes occur with any frequency. Drug-induced mania must occupy the first three places on any differential diagnostic list. The immunologically based syndromes can be accorded fourth place. The other etiologies are less commonly encountered, and when affective instability does occur during the clinical course of CNS infections, trauma, or metabolic derangement, it is usually not difficult to recognize what is happening. What to do about it may be another matter, but in this book we are concentrating on diagnostic issues. Accordingly, we will devote relatively more space to the drug-induced and immunologic forms of secondary mania. Reviews of this topic are provided in the Krauthammer and Klerman article (1978) and in Stasiek and Zetin (1985).

Two more comments are in order before we turn to the syndromes themselves. We have the impression that the mental status examination itself is relatively *less* useful in alerting clinicians to the presence of a secondary manic episode when compared with secondary depressive episodes. Those impairments of arousal, orientation, concentration, and attention focusing that are clues to the presence of encephalopathy or structural brain disease are more difficult to establish reliably during the examination of manic patients. Moreover, mania itself can produce these cognitive impairments (Hanes, 1912). Treatment response to psychopharmacologic agents such as lithium and antipsychotic drugs is another feature that fails to distinguish primary from secondary manic episodes (Hale and Donaldson, 1982). This is good news for the

*See Chapter 5 for a discussion of our terminology. In brief, we will use terms such as "secondary mania" in this book to denote manic episodes that occur during the course of metabolic or neurologic dysfunction of various etiologies.

**Table 6.1**
Medical and Neurologic Syndromes Associated with Secondary Mania

| | |
|---|---|
| Drugs and toxins | Immunologic |
| *Corticosteroids*[a] | *Systemic lupus erythematosus* |
| *Dopamine agonists* | *Multiple sclerosis* |
| Decongestants | Endocrine |
| Bronchodilators | *Hyperthyroidism* |
| Alpha-methyldopa | Cushing's disease |
| Amphetamines | Brain tumor |
| Methylphenidate | Multiple cell types and anatomy |
| Cocaine | Metabolic |
| *Tricyclic antidepressants* | Hemodialysis |
| L-tryptophan/monoamine oxidase inhibitor | Postoperative state |
| Flutamide | $B_{12}$ deficiency |
| *Trazadone* | Calcium infusion |
| Cyclobenzaprine | Hypoxia |
| Monoamine oxidase inhibitors | Infection |
| Thyroid hormone | Neurosyphilis |
| Procarbazine | Cryptococcosis |
| Bromide | Influenza |
| Phencyclidine | Fever |
| Metoclopramide | St. Louis type A encephalitis |
| Cyclosporine | AIDS |
| Procyclidine | CNS degenerative disease |
| Digitalis | Spinocerebellar atrophy |
| Reserpine withdrawal | Epilepsy |
| Antidepressant withdrawal | Stroke |
| Baclofen | |
| Niridazole | |
| Alprazolam | |
| CNS trauma | |

[a]Italicized entities are discussed in the text.

clinician who must manage such patients, but it makes it even more difficult in those relatively rare instances where the etiology of a manic episode is genuinely in doubt.

## DRUG- OR TOXIN-INDUCED MANIA

A 26-year-old woman is followed in endocrinology clinic for systemic lupus erythematosus, complicated by arthritis and nephritis. Recently, her joint symptoms worsened and her erythrocyte sedimentation rate rose to 80. Her alternate-day prednisone regimen was increased to 80 mg daily. Mania supervened.

The list of drugs in Table 6.1 that have been reported to induce the manic syndrome is a long one (for a review of drugs that can mimic psychiatric syndromes, see Medical Letter, 1986). With a few exceptions, however, the entire list can be reduced to two categories of drugs—corticosteroids, and drugs that up-regulate catecholamine transmission in the central nervous system.

When the use of corticosteroids in large numbers of medical patients is reviewed, the incidence of drug-related psychiatric syndromes is variably reported between 13% and 62%, with a weighted average of 27.6% (Lewis and Smith, 1983). Most of these reactions are mild and do not require either treatment or discontinuation of the steroid medication. Although many reports describe depression and dysphoric side effects, we have been impressed (along with Lewis and Smith, 1983, and Glaser, 1953) that psychomotor acceleration, mild euphoria, and decreased need for sleep are so common as to be the rule early in a steroid course. These hypomanic features during the first week of the treatment require clinical attention, since progression to the full manic syndrome can occur. There is evidence that these hypomanic drug reactions are dose-dependent. They may occur at rates approaching 70% for patients who receive the equivalent of 60 mg of prednisone per day, but may be unobtrusive or nonexistent for patients on lower doses (Boston Collaborative Drug Surveillance Program, 1972; Cade *et al.*, 1973). The depressive side effects of these drugs generally appear later in the course of their administration or during the pharmacologic taper. We again remark upon the clinical paradox that acutely administered exogenous corticosteroids tend to make patients feel hyperalert and accelerated, whereas Cushing's syndrome more typically presents with feelings of depression. The mechanisms involved in this disparity are not known. In addition, we have the strong clinical impression that mania associated with exogenous steroid administration is a marker for underlying vulnerability to affective disturbance on the part of the patient. There is no evidence to support such a contention at this time, however.

In addition to corticosteroids, it appears that any drug that can directly or indirectly increase central catecholamine (and perhaps indoleamine) transmission can also induce manic features (Harsch, 1984; Shader, 1972; Ryback and Schwab, 1971; Bunnet *et al.*, 1970; Goff, 1985). This includes antidepressants of all types, antiparkinsonian drugs, decongestants and some bronchodilators, and all types of psychostimulants. Apparently patients need to have no previous history of affective disorders to experience a drug-related manic episode, although those who "switch" from depression to mania while on tricyclics may have an underlying bipolar diathesis. Typically the switch process to mania or the development of drug-related manic features appears within 3–14 days of drug initiation.

In looking again at the drugs listed in Table 6.1, it is interesting that administration of tricyclic and nontricyclic antidepressants has been associated with secondary mania, but so has the *withdrawal* of tricyclic antidepressants.

This represents yet another clinical paradox without a definite explanation, although an imbalance in alterations of cholinergic and monoaminergic receptor systems has been proposed (Dilsaver and Greden, 1984).

## Demographics

The drug- and toxin-induced secondary manias occur in heterogeneous subpopulation of patients, so no generalizations can be made. With the exception of young adults who are "occult" psychostimulant abusers, most of these subpopulations are readily identified: parkinsonian patients, affective-disorder patients who have been prescribed antidepressants, and patients with immunologic diseases receiving corticosteroids.

## Clinical History

With the exception of some psychostimulant drug abusers, the clinical history of drug usage is readily obtained. Upon seeing a new manic patient, the examiner should immediately wonder, "Could this patient be taking corticosteroids or any drugs that alter catecholamine turnover or transmission?" When diagnostic errors are made, they are usually errors of omitting this conceptual step, as opposed to an inability to elicit the information from the patient.

## Psychotropic Drug Interactions

Antipsychotics. The safety of antipsychotic medication in drug-induced mania is limited only by the precariousness of the underlying medical illness. Dopamine *blockade* makes neurophysiologic sense in a syndrome that may be attributable to up-regulation of catecholamine transmission.

Lithium. Lithium is generally safe in drug-induced mania and may be administered prophylactically to patients who require episodic courses of steroids. This medication should be avoided in parkinsonian patients if possible, since lithium has dopamine receptor-blocking properties of its own and may worsen extrapyramidal features.

## Mental Status Examination

There is no evidence that mental status findings are useful in distinguishing drug-induced mania from the mania of bipolar disorders.

### General Medical Examination

Document blood pressure, heart rate, and rhythm. These may rise to dangerous levels in some cases of adrenergic drug overdosage.

### Neurological Examination

Cranial Nerves. Nystagmus, if prominent or persistent, may indicate adrenergic drug use. Subhyaloid hemorrhages may appear in amphetamine abuse complicated by subarachnoid hemorrhage and may be seen easily on ophthalmoscopic examination.

Motor. Significant postural tremor or limb discoordination favors drug etiology, as does the presence of choreiform movement disorder.

Reflex. Diffuse, symmetric hyperreflexia may be seen in mania of all types and is probably not helpful in making etiologic distinctions.

### Laboratory and Imaging

Corticosteroids. Serum and urinary assays for cortisol and hydroxy- and ketosteroids may be done but are not usually necessary in assessing drug-induced mania.

Adrenergic Drugs. Levels of tricyclic antidepressants including amitriptyline, imipramine, desipramine, and nortriptyline may be measured in serum. Amphetamines may be measured in urine.

## IMMUNOLOGIC DISEASE-INDUCED MANIA

A 26-year-old woman is followed in endocrinology clinic for systemic lupus erythematosus, complicated by arthritis and nephritis. Recently, her joint symptoms worsened and her erythrocyte sedimentation rate rose to 80. Her alternate-day prednisone regimen was increased to 80 mg daily. Mania supervened.

*Note:* If this vignette sounds similar to that which introduced the previous section, it's because they are identical. We haven't said yet which pathophysiology applies; corticosteroids or lupus.

Only two immunologically based diseases come under consideration for association with secondary mania: systemic lupus erythematosus (SLE), and multiple sclerosis (MS). In both diseases, clinicians seek such an association much more often than they find it.

## Systemic Lupus Erythematosus

SLE is one of a family of collagen vascular diseases that tend to affect women more commonly than men. Onset is typically during early adult life, during the years when first manic episodes of bipolar disorders are also likely to occur. The most common *initial* symptoms and signs of SLE tend to be arthritis, arthralgias, and cutaneous disorders, as opposed to neurologic or behavioral symptoms (Estes and Christian, 1971), although it is clear that SLE can present first with symptoms or signs referable to the central nervous system. The disease is currently diagnosed according to a set of criteria including both clinical features and laboratory abnormalities (Table 6.2) (Tan *et al.*, 1982). Any patient who meets four of the 11 criteria has the disease by stipulation.

A variety of immunologic laboratory tests are now available to assist the clinician in diagnosing or monitoring SLE. The diagnostic sensitivity (rate of false negatives) and specificity (rate of false positives) of four are presented in Table 6.3 (Calabrese, 1984).

The *antinuclear antibodies* are a family of circulating autoantibodies against components of the cell nucleus. A peripheral pattern around the nuclear membrane is associated with antibodies to native DNA (N-DNA). A speckled pattern, with staining material spread throughout the nuclear material, indicates antibodies to an extractable nucleus antigen. The nucleolar pattern is caused by a reaction with messenger RNA. The presence of *anti-N-DNA* (or anti-double-stranded DNA) is very specific for SLE, although not all SLE patients are positive. The titer of this antibody often correlates with disease activity. The *anti-Sm* is one of several antibodies to extractable nuclear antigens that may appear in the course of the disease (anti-RNP, anti-SSA, and anti-SS-B are others). Anti-Sm is specific for SLE, but the others are more often positive in other connective-tissue diseases. Three tests that are not specific but that are useful in monitoring disease activity include the presence of circulating immune complexes, depressed serum complement, and the erythrocyte sedimentation rate. The LE cell test is little used at the present time. All of these tests are performed on serum.

Patients with SLE develop mental status and behavioral abnormalities during the course of their illness at a very high rate (Bresnihan, 1982; Feinglass *et al.*, 1976; Ganz *et al.*, 1972). One can expect 20–40% of such patients to develop behavioral disturbance at some time during the course of illness, which is attributable to CNS involvement by the immunologic disease. Other behavioral disturbances may be attributable to side effects of corticosteroid, quinacrine, and antimetabolite medications. Still other disturbances of mentation occur in the setting of metabolic disturbances induced by the lupus, such as in the encephalopathy associated with uremia. This distinction between behavioral disturbances associated with primary CNS involvement by SLE and drug-induced

**Table 6.2**
The 1982 Revised Criteria for Diagnosis of Systemic Lupus Erythematosus

| Criterion | Definition |
|---|---|
| 1. Malar rash | Fixed erythema, flat or raised, over the malar eminences tending to spare the nasolabial folds |
| 2. Discoid rash | Erythematous raised patches with adherent keratotic scaling and follicular plugging; atrophic scarring may occur in older lesions |
| 3. Photosensitivity | Skin rash as a result of unusual reaction to sunlight, by patient history or physician observation |
| 4. Oral ulcers | Oral or nasopharyngeal ulceration, usually painless, observed by a physician |
| 5. Arthritis | Nonerosive arthritis involving two or more peripheral joints, characterized by tenderness, swelling, or effusion |
| 6. Serositis | Pleuritis—convincing history of pleuritic pain or rub heard by a physician or evidence of pleural effusion—*or* pericarditis—documented by EKG or rub or evidence of pericardial effusion |
| 7. Renal disorder | Persistent proteinuria greater than 0.5 g day or greater than 3+ if quantitation not performed, *or* cellular casts—may be red cell, hemoglobin, granular, tubular, or mixed |
| 8. Neurologic disorder | Seizures—in the absence of offending drugs or known metabolic derangements, e.g., uremia, ketoacidosis, or electrolyte imbalance—*or* psychosis—in the absence of offending drugs or known metabolic derangements, e.g., uremia ketoacidosis or electrolyte imbalance |
| 9. Hematologic disorder | Hemolytic anemia, with reticulocytosis, *or* leukopenia, less than $4000/mm^3$ total on two or more occasions, *or* lymphopenia, less than $1500/mm^3$ on two or more occasions, *or* thrombocytopenia, less than $100{,}000/mm^3$ in the absence of offending drugs |
| 10. Immunologic disorder | Positive LE cell preparation, *or* anti-DNA: antibody to native DNA in abnormal titer, *or* anti-Sm: presence of antibody to Sm nuclear antigen, *or* false-positive serologic test for syphilis known to be positive for at least 6 months and confirmed by *Treponema pallidum* immoilization of fluorescent treponemal antibody absorption test |
| 11. Antinuclear antibody | An abnormal titer of antinuclear antibody by immunofluorescence or an equivalent assay at any point in time and in the absence of drugs known to be associated with "drug-induced lupus" syndrome |

**Table 6.3**
Sensitivity and Specificity of Serum Tests for SLE

| Test | Sensitivity | Specificity |
|---|---|---|
| ANA titer | 0.990 | 0.690 |
| Anti-N-DNA titer | 0.569 | 0.993 |
| Anti-Sm titer | 0.220 | 0.999 |
| LE cell | 0.704 | 0.946 |

or metabolically induced changes in mentation is of great clinical significance. Major therapeutic decisions may rest on this issue, and the stakes may be high. Unfortunately, there is no clear consensus on the reliable determination of CNS SLE activity. One of the difficulties may be that we are not really certain of the mechanism by which SLE may affect brain function. There is some evidence in favor of a microvascular neuropathologic mechanism in CNS lupus, and other evidence suggesting a more direct antineuronal antibody response. It is possible that more than one pathophysiology can occur.

Although we are including SLE within the chapter on mania, it should be recognized from the start that no specific psychiatric syndrome can be expected among SLE patients. Affective disturbances, both manic and depressed, may be seen along with a spectrum of psychiatric states and a variety of other psychoneurotic features. In some cases, the psychiatric disturbance seems clearly to have been unrelated to fluctuations in the underlying SLE, but in many other cases these signs have been evidence of CNS vasculitis and inflammation. When CNS vasculitis involvement from SLE has been present, other more neurologic signs have often been present: seizures, tremor or incoordination, and hemiparesis, or long tract signs. A rising ESR or falling serum complement may be seen. The mental status in such patients has often been characterized by disorientation, impaired concentration, and failure of verbal learning.

We must close this discussion of affective syndromes associated with lupus cerebritis by observing that they are much rarer in our experience than seems to be the case at other medical centers. When the differential diagnostic issue arises between lupus affective disorder versus drug- or metabolically induced affective disorder, we have almost always found the latter. We do not doubt that a true lupus affective disorder can occur, but clinicians should favor drug or metabolic etiologies when in doubt.

## Demographics

Lupus demonstrates a mean age of onset of approximately 30 years, and women outnumber men with the disease by a ratio of 3:1 or 4:1.

## Clinical History

As we have mentioned, the difficult clinical issue for mental health practitioners is not usually mistaking the first symptom of lupus for a psychiatric disorder (although this can happen) but in discerning subsequent behavioral disturbances as related to CNS lupus, to drugs, to metabolic problems associated with the disease, or to psychological difficulties. We provide no easy answers here.

At initial presentation the disease is protean, but typically there is a relapsing/remitting history of signs and symptoms from Table 6.2. Arthraglias, arthritis, and skin lesions are particularly common early in the disease course. Such patients are difficult for medical practitioners, and the diagnosis is often not made until several years after disease onset.

At the time of a behavioral disturbance in someone who may have SLE, one should attempt to obtain a clinical history concerning extra-CNS manifestations of disease activity. Have there been new joint symptoms, myalgias, or other constitutional symptoms? Although CNS lupus may occur without concurrent exacerbation of extra-CNS disease activity, they may be associated. Has the patient had headaches? Although nonspecific, we have been impressed that most patients with behavioral disturbances associated with CNS lupus have had a headache prodrome. This headache is often described as throbbing, migrainelike, but more chronic in course.

The issue of recent drug changes must also be classified in the clinical history. Increase in corticosteroid dosing to 40 mg/day of prednisone equivalent or more for several weeks prior to onset of affective disturbance is very suspicious for steroid-induced affective disturbances. Quinacrine is also prescribed for SLE and has been reported less commonly to be associated with confusional and maniclike states.

## Psychotropic Drug Interaction

Corticosteroids and quinine derivatives have both been associated with affective disturbances and confusional states. See our previous discussion of corticosteroid-induced mania.

## Mental Status Examination

When a mental status change is produced by lupus cerebritis, the MSE typically shows evidence of delirium or encephalopathy along with whatever affective features may be present.

**Arousal.** Disturbance of arousal is probably the most sensitive mental status function when lupus cerebritis occurs. The arousal disturbance represents a disturbance with a broad spectrum of severity, ranging from stupor and coma to much milder impairments of the ability to sustain concentration. Mental status tests that require sustained concentration should be administered: serial digit repetitions, alternate response tests, tests that involve writing.

Orientation. May be impaired in moderate to severe cerebritis, but these tests are probably not of great sensitivity.

Verbal Learning. Cooperation is always a question during a manic episode, but the examiner may attempt the ten-word list described in Chapter 3. Serious deficits may be consistent with encephalopathy secondary to cerebritis.

Affective Symptoms. There is no evidence that the quality of the manic (or depressive) symptomatology itself is unusual in lupus cerebritis.

## General Medical Examination

The examiner checks for features listed in Table 6.1. *Skin:* Discoid or malar rash; photosensitivity or sun-induced rash. *HEENT:* Oral ulcers. *Musculoskeletal:* Small-joint arthritis. *Chest:* Pleuritis or pleural rub. *Cardiac:* Friction rub.

## Neurological Examination

Stroke, seizures, choreiform movement disorders, and peripheral neuropathic syndromes may occur during the course of central or peripheral nervous system involvement by lupus. It is not certain that the neuropathologic mechanisms involved in these neurologic syndromes are the same as those involved in the lupus behavioral disorders. Since at least the CNS neurologic disorders are reliable evidence of involvement by the disease, however, they should be considered.

Motor. Hemispheric motor syndromes may be seen in lupus cerebritis. Look for subtle evidence of upper motor neuron pattern weakness—pronator drift or unilateral slowing of fine motor movements. Cerebellar systems dysfunction may also be present. One should check for postural tremor; incoordination on finger-to-nose or heel-to-shin testing; gait ataxia; ability to perform the Romberg maneuver.

Reflex. Symmetric hyperreflexia may be an early sign of cerebritis. The presence of pathologic reflexes (Babinski sign, Hoffman's sign, release signs) may also be suggestive of CNS disease.

Sensory. Patients with SLE and related diseases may develop peripheral neuropathic syndromes, especially mononeuropathy multiplex. Patchy hyperpathia or dysesthesia in the distribution of peripheral nerves should be sought.

### Laboratory and Imaging

Serologic diagnostic tests have been discussed earlier and are listed in Table 6.3. The following tests may be useful in distinguishing an acute exacerbation, but no laboratory test is definitive.

Serum. Rising or elevated ESR. The degree of change from a previous baseline may be more important than the absolute level. Falling or depressed serum complement is also useful.

Urinalysis. New proteinuria, hematuria.

Cerebrospinal Fluid. A variety of CSF abnormalities have been reported in lupus cerebritis including: (1) mononuclear pleocytosis; (2) hypoglycorrhea; (3) elevated total protein; (4) elevated IgG (>10% of total protein, or >15% of albumin); (5) oligoclonal banding of IgG. It appears that more than 50% of patients with active CNS lupus will demonstrate one or more of these abnormalities, making the lumbar puncture a very important test for this clinical problem. Unfortunately, a normal CSF does not exclude the diagnosis of CNS lupus.

Head CT Scan. Evidence of diffuse inflammation with contrast enhancement.

EEG. Slowing and disorganization of the EEG are quite sensitive to CNS lupus but are not very specific. The EEG is most helpful in distinguishing lupus psychosis from steroid psychosis, in which it should be normal.

## Multiple Sclerosis

MS is also listed as an immune-mediated disease that may occasionally mimic or be associated with a manic syndrome (Mapelli and Ramelli, 1981; Kwentus *et al.*, 1986). There is also an epidemiologic report, indicating that bipolar affective disorder occurs with a greater frequency than expected among patients with MS (Schiffer *et al.*, 1986). The diagnosis may be worth considering in young women with neurologic complaints such as difficulty walking, numbness and tingling, monocular blindness, or difficulty with urination. The evaluation of patients for potential MS is described in Chapter 5.

## ENDOCRINE DISEASE AND MANIA

There are scattered case reports of manic syndromes occurring in association with elevated levels of serum T4 or with the onset of clinical hyperthyroidism (Villani and Weitzel, 1979; Corn and Checkley, 1983; Weinberg and Katzell, 1977). There is at least one case report of a manic psychosis that supervened 4 days after the initiation of therapy for hypothyroidism with exogenous thyroxine (Josephson and MacKenzie, 1979). We have seen another example of mania after initiation of thyroid hormone replacement, and we suspect that it occurs more commonly than would be judged from the literature. In our judgment, however, early clinical hyperthyroidism is more likely to be mistaken for an anxiety disorder than for mania, and we have placed our detailed discussions of the evaluation of hyperthyroidism in Chapter 7.

There is at least one case report of bipolar disorder occurring in association with undiagnosed Cushing's syndrome (Kane and Keeler, 1962). Since depressive symptomatology seems much more commonly associated with this endocrinologic disturbance, we have placed our more detailed discussion of the diagnostic evaluation of Cushing's syndrome in Chapter 5.

## CNS TUMOR AND MANIA

A 40-year-old woman had worked for 20 years as a clerical assistant, with an exemplary work record. She had no history of psychopathology and no family history of affective disturbance. At the age of 40, she developed her first manic episode, which was successfully treated with haloperidol. Her medical and neurological examinations on admission general were recorded as "normal." Because of her relatively late age of onset for a first manic episode, a head CT scan was obtained, which showed a large, enhancing tumor distorting the right lateral ventricle. On repeated and more careful neurological examination, she was noted to have a left pronator drift and clonus at the left ankle.

The scenario in which an occult brain tumor *presents* as mania is rare. Krauthammer and Klerman (1978) reviewed three such case reports, and Stasiek and Zetin (1985) added two more. Greenberg and Brown (1985) have since described one additional patient with lung carcinoma metastatic to right diencephalon, with secondary mania, and Binder (1983) has reported a woman with recurrent mania which resolved after removal of a right-hemisphere meningioma.

When these case reports are reviewed, it seems to have been the case that the mental status examination did not provide the important diagnostic clues. The patients demonstrated manic features on the emotional portion of the mental status examination, and cognitive testing tended to be either difficult to do or unrewarding. In almost each case, however, some subtle but definite abnormalities were present within other sections of the neurologic examination. Most often these findings were within the motor or reflex portions of the examination and included tremor, ataxia, reflex asymmetry, and unilateral pathologic reflexes. The majority of these cases revealed tremors that involved either high-brainstem or right-hemispheric structures and probably produced manic symptomatology by interfering either with brainstem amine systems or with right-hemispheric regulation of emotion. No particular tumor cell type was in evidence. In addition, clinicians were alerted by the absence of past psychiatric history or family psychiatric histories in these patients and by the relatively late age of onset for a manic disorder (i.e., in the fifth or sixth decades).

## Demographics

First onset of a manic episode after age 35 or manic episodes occurring in the setting of a negative family history for affective disorders are warning signs for the presence of secondary mania. Brain tumors in adults demonstrate an incidence rate of approximately 8 per 100,000 person-years, both for primary and metastatic tumors. The most common primary tumors are gliomas of various grades, meningiomas, pituitary adenomas, and neurinomas. The most common metastatic tumors to brain are lung, breast, renal, and melanomas. Gliomas, neurinomas, and adenomas are more common among women. Generalizations are risky, but most of these tumors tend to be hemispheric in location and to demonstrate clinical onset during the fourth decade or later.

## Clinical History

Brain tumors, whether primary or metastatic, produce variable signs and symptoms, depending on their cell type and location. The fundamental rule from clinical neurology is that tumors produce gradually progressive neurologic complaints or findings. Common complaints referable to hemispheric tumors include headache, nausea, disequilibrium, personality and affective change, focal weakness, and seizures.

*Clinical Rule No. 6.1:* Any gradually progressive neurologic complaint or finding is due to a tumor, until such time as a better explanation can be found.

## Psychotropic Drug Interactions

None. Remember that a therapeutic response of mania to lithium or antipsychotic medication proves nothing about the etiology of the mania.

### Mental Status Examination

Not generally helpful, primarily because it is difficult to perform carefully in manic patients. Manic patients by definition have defects in attention and concentration but should be generally intact in areas of orientation, language, learning, and calculations. Significant defects in these latter functions might suggest neurologic or medical disease, but clinical judgment and experience must temper such conclusions.

### General Physical Examination

Not generally helpful in primary tumors, which rarely metastasize *out* of the central nervous system. Stigmata of primary malignancies involving skin, breast, and lungs are worth pursuing.

### Neurological Examination

This is the checkpoint that appears to have been the most useful in picking up CNS mass lesions among manic patients. The brainstem tumors cause subtle but definite impairment in cerebellar system functions or in cranial nerve functions. The hemispheric tumors produce reflex abnormalities or asymmetric weakness of upper motor neuron pattern.

### Laboratory and Imaging

At the present time the head CT scan probably remains the imaging test of first choice when CNS tumor is suspected. The majority of tumors that can be imaged are seen on the uncontrasted scan, so it is not always necessary to order the scan with contrast. We suggest that the clinician's degree of suspicion decide whether to obtain both a contrasted and uncontrasted scan. If the neurologic signs are soft and suspicion is low, a scan without contrast may serve as a satisfactory screening test. A magnetic resonance image is more sensitive to brainstem pathology and should probably be the initial test when cranial nerve findings are present.

## METABOLIC-INDUCED MANIA

Mania in association with metabolic derangement or delirium is not the same thing as "delirious mania." The latter term denotes the profile of cognitive deficits, especially in attention and arousal, which may occur in the course of a manic episode. We are using the term "metabolic-induced mania" to denote those syndromes of significant metabolic derangement in which manic features appear. These are really metabolic encephalopathies with admixed manic features. Table 6.1 lists five such metabolic encephalopathies that have been reported to produce manic signs or symptoms, but we suspect there are many more. Any metabolic derangement that depresses the function of enough neurons through the hemispheres may produce a disinhibited state vaguely resembling mania. This rarely poses a diagnostic problem for mental health clinicians, although one should be alert to the manic patient with concomitant renal failure or hypoxic lung disease. All of these patients should have coexistent impairments of attention, concentrations, and verbal learning ability.

## INFECTION-INDUCED MANIA

As in case of the metabolic manias, most of the reports of infection-induced mania have described patients with admixed manic and encephalopathic features. For example, Thienhaus and Khosla (1984) described a 63-year-old man who developed his first affective episode in the setting of urinary incontinence, disorientation to time and place, and a global block in verbal learning. On evaluation, he was found to be suffering from meningeal cryptococcosis. Neurosyphilis is another worrisome infection in this group that has a reputation for generating accelerated and euphoric behaviors (see Chapter 5 for review of the diagnostic evaluation). Mapelli and Bellelli have reported a 34-year-old man who developed manic features in the setting of treatment with penicillin G for neurosyphilis. However, this patient had telling neurologic difficulties including focal seizures and aphasia. This report confirms our clinical experience that most patients with mania secondary to CNS infection have discernible neurologic, cognitive, or systemic signs which provide palpable clues, assuming that the patient is examined.

There is a somewhat unsettling case report, however, of a young woman who appears to have developed mania as the initial CNS feature of AIDS (Gabel *et al.*, 1986). The manic patient reported in this study appears to have had a normal neurologic examination, relatively intact cognition, and unremarkable neurodiagnostic testing including EEG, CSF analysis, and head CT scan. Only her evolving clinical course made the HIV manifest. Clinicians may have to consider sending serum for HIV antibody liters during the evaluation of manic patients.

## EPILEPSY-INDUCED MANIA

As noted in the previous chapter, the affective syndromes associated with the various forms of epilepsy have been much more poorly studied than the psychoses (see Chapter 8 for more detailed consideration of the workup for epilepsy). In those studies of temporal lobe focus epilepsy in which affective disorders are considered, mania is but rarely mentioned. Krauthammer and Klerman (1978) refer to a single such case, and that person had experienced widespread CNS trauma from subarachnoid hemorrhage and neurosurgery. Hurwitz *et al.* (1985) have reported a man with partial complex seizures and bilateral EEG foci who experienced prolonged hypomanic behavior after right hemisphere seizures. Once again, however, it does not sound as if either of these cases provided diagnostic puzzles for mental health clinicians. It has not been our clinical experience that patients with active temporal lobe seizures are easily mistaken for bipolar patients.

## TRAUMA-INDUCED MANIA

The occurrence of mania after relatively severe brain injury is a subject that has just recently begun to receive clinical research attention (Shukla *et al.*, 1987; Starkstein *et al.*, 1987). It is apparent that at least a small number of patients may develop mania within the first 3 years after brain injury and that such a development is more likely if the injury has involved anterior deep limbic system structures or right-hemisphere structures. Interestingly, some of these patients have family histories positive for depressive–affective disturbances, as if an interaction between trauma and genetic vulnerability were a prerequisite. The history of trauma was readily apparent in the reported cases. Several of the patients had posttraumatic epilepsy, and most had abnormal head CT scans.

## CNS DEGENERATIVE DISEASE AND MANIA

There is one report of two patients with coexistent spinocerebellar degeneration and mania (Yadalam *et al.*, 1985), but from this it is difficult to draw any useful clinical conclusions.

## STROKE AND MANIA

There are several reports of patients who developed mania quite soon after stroke (Jampala and Abrams, 1987; Cohen and Niska, 1980). In most of these cases, the stroke involved subarachnoid hemorrhage, or intracerebral hemorrhage, so extensive and diffuse cerebral damage was likely experienced. None of these patients presented diagnostic dilemmas for the psychiatric clinicians, although they often proved difficult to treat.

## REFERENCES


Binder, R. L. Neurologically silent brain tumors in psychiatric hospital admissions: Three cases and a review. *J. Clin. Psychiatry,* 1983, **44,** 94–97.

Boston Collaborative Drug Surveillance Program. Acute adverse reactions to prednisone in relation to dosage. *Clin. Pharmacol. Ther.,* 1972, **13,** 694–698.

Bresnihan, B. CNS lupus. *Clin. Rheum. Dis.,* 1982, **8,** 183–195.

Bunney, W. E. Jr., Murphy, D. L., Goodwin, F. K., and Borge, G. F. The switch process from depression to mania: Relationship to drugs which alter brain amines. *Lancet,* 1970, **1,** 1022–1027.

Cade, R., Spooner, G., Schlein, E., Pickering, M., De Quesada, A., Holcomb, A., Juncos, L., Richard, G., Shires, D., Levin, D., Hackett, R., Free, J., Hunt, R., and Fregly, M. Comparison of azathioprine, prednisone, and heparin alone or combined in treating lupus nephritis. *Nephron,* 1973, **10,** 37–56.

Calabrese, L. H. Diagnosis of systemic lupus erythematosus. *Postgrad Med.,* 1984, **75**(7), 103–112.

Cohen, M. R., and Niska, R. W. Localized right cerebral hemisphere dysfunction and recurrent mania. *Am. J. Psychiatry,* 1980, **137,** 847–848.

Corn, T. H., and Checkley, S. A. A case of recurrent mania with recurrent hyperthyroidism. *Br. J. Psychiatry,* 1983, **143,** 74–76.

*Diagnostic and Statistical Manual of Mental Disorders,* 3d ed., revised. Washington, DC: American Psychiatric Association, 1987.

Dilsaver, S. C., and Greden, J. F. Antidepressant withdrawal-induced activation (hypomania and mania): Mechanism and theoretical significance. *Brain Res.,* 1984, **319,** 29–48.

Estes, D., and Christian, C. L. The natural history of systemic lupus erythematosus by prospective analysis. *Medicine,* 1971, **50,** 85–95.

Feinglass, E. J., Arnett, F. C., Dorsch, C. A., Zizic, T. M., and Stevens, M. B. Neuropsychiatric manifestations of systemic lupus erythematosus: Diagnosis, clinical spectrum, and relationship to other features of the disease. *Medicine,* 1976, **55,** 323–339.

Gabel, R. H., Barnard, N., Norko, M., and O'Connell, R. A. AIDS presenting as mania. *Compr. Psychiatry,* 1986, **27,** 251–254.

Ganz, V. H., Gurland, B. J., Deming, W. E., and Fisher, B. The study of the psychiatric symptoms of systemic lupus erythematosus: A biometric study. *Psychosom. Med.,* 1972, **34,** 207–220.

Glaser, G. H. Psychotic reactions induced by corticotropin (ACTH) and cortisone. *Psychosom. Med.,* 1953, **15,** 280–291.

Goff, D. C. Two cases of hypomania following the addition of L-tryptophan to a monoamine oxidase inhibitor. *Am. J. Psychiatry,* 1985, **142,** 1487–1488.

Greenberg, D. B., and Brown, G. L. Single case study: Mania resulting from brain stem tumor. *J. Nerv. Ment. Dis.,* 1985, **173,** 434–436.

Hale, M. S., and Donaldson, J. O. Lithium carbonate in the treatment of organic brain syndrome. *J. Nerv. Ment. Dis.,* 1982, **170,** 362–365.

Hanes, E. L. Acute delirium in psychiatric practice, with special reference to so-called acute delirious mania (collapse delirium). *J. Nerv. Ment. Dis.,* 1912, **39,** 236–250.

Harsch, H. H. Mania in two patients following cyclobenzaprine. *Psychosomatics,* 1984, **25,** 791–793.

Hurwitz, T. A., Wada, J. A., Kosaka, B. D., and Strauss, E. H. Cerebral organization of affect suggested by temporal lobe seizures. *Neurology,* 1985, **35,** 1335–1337.

Jampala, V. C., and Abrams, R. Mania secondary to left and right hemisphere damage. *Am. J. Psychiatry,* 1983, **140,** 1197–1199.

Josephson, A. M., and MacKenzie, T. B. Appearance of manic psychosis following rapid normalization of thyroid status. *Am. J. Psychiatry,* 1979, **136,** 846–847.

Kane, F. J., and Keeler, M. H. Mania seen with undiagnosed Cushing's syndrome. *Am. J. Psychiatry,* 1962, **119,** 267–268.

Krauthammer,, C., and Klerman, G. L. Secondary mania: Manic syndromes associated with antecedent physical illness or drugs. *Arch. Gen. Psychiatry,* 1978, **35,** 1333–1339.

Kwentus, J. A., Hart, R. P., Calabrese, V., and Hekmati, A. Mania as a symptom of multiple sclerosis. *Psychosomatics,* 1986, **27,** 729–731.

Lewis, D. A., and Smith, R. E. Steroid-induced psychiatric syndromes: A report of 14 cases and a review of the literature. *J. Affective Disord.,* 1983, **5,** 319–322.

Mapelli, G., and Bellelli, T. Secondary mania. *Arch. Gen. Psychiatry,* 1982, **39,** 743 (letter).

Mapelli, G., and Ramelli, E. Manic syndrome associated with multiple sclerosis: "Secondary mania?" *Acta Psychiatr. Belg.,* 1981, **81,** 337–349.

Medical Letter. Drugs that cause psychiatric symptoms. *Med. Lett. Drugs Ther.,* 1986, **28,** 81–86.

*Mental Disorders: Glossary and Guide to Their Classification in Accordance with the Ninth Revision of the International Classification of Diseases.* Geneva: World Health Organization, 1978.

Ryback, R. S., and Schwab, R. S. Manic response to levodopa therapy, report of a case. *N. Engl. J. Med.,* 1971, **285,** 788–789.

Schiffer, R. B., Wineman, N. M., and Weitkamp, L. R. Association between bipolar affective disorder and multiple sclerosis. *Am. J. Psychiatry,* 1986, **143,** 94–95.

Shader, R. I. *Psychiatric Complications of Medical Drugs.* New York: Raven Press, 1972.

Shukla, S., Cook, B. L., Mukherjee, S., Godwin, C., and Miller, M. G. Mania following head trauma. *Am. J. Psychiatry,* 1987, **144,** 93–96.

Starkstein, S. E., Pearlson, G. D., Boston, J., and Robinson, R. G. Mania after brain injury: A controlled study of causative factors. *Arch. Neurol.,* 1987, **44,** 1069–1073.

Stasiek, C., and Zetin, M. Organic manic disorders. *Psychosomatics,* 1985, **26,** 394–402.

Tan, E. M., Cohen, A. S., Fries, J. F., Masi, A. T., McShane, D. J., Rothfield, N. F., Schaller, J. G., Talal, N., and Winchester, R. J. The 1982 revised criteria for the classification of systemic lupus erythematosus. *Arthritis Rheum.,* 1982, **25,** 1271–1277.

Thienhaus, O. J., and Khosla, N. Meningeal cryptococcosis misdiagnosed as a manic episode. *Am. J. Psychiatry,* 1984, **141,** 1459–1460.

Villani, S., and Weitzel, W. D. Secondary mania. *Arch. Gen. Psychiatry,* 1979, **36,** 1031 (letter).

Weinberg, A. D., and Katzell, T. D. Thyroid and adrenal function among psychiatric patients. *Lancet,* 1977, **1,** 1104–1105.

Yadalam, K. G., Jain, A. K., and Simpson, G. M. Mania in two sisters with similar cerebellar disturbance. *Am. J. Psychiatry,* 1985, **142,** 1067–1069.

# 7

# Anxiety Syndrome

### DSM-III-R Disorders

*Panic Disorders with and without Agoraphobia.* The essential features of these disorders are recurrent panic attacks, i.e., discrete periods of intense fear or discomfort. The panic attacks usually last minutes or, more rarely, hours. They are accompanied by associated somatic symptoms, such as dyspnea, palpitations, diaphoresis, tingling, and others.

*Phobic Disorders* (social phobia, simple phobia, agoraphobia). The essential feature of these disorders is a persistent fear of situations or stimuli, which is recognized by the patient as excessive or unreasonable.

*Generalized Anxiety Disorder.* The essential feature of this disorder is unrealistic or excessive anxiety and worry about two or more life circumstances during 6 months or longer. Symptoms of motor tension and autonomic hyperactivity commonly accompany this disorder.

### ICD-9 Disorders

*Anxiety States.* Various combinations of physical and mental manifestations of anxiety, not attributable to real danger and occurring either in attacks or as a persisting state. The anxiety is usually diffuse and may extend to panic. Other neurotic features such as obsessional or hysterical symptoms may be present but do not dominate the clinical picture.

The anxiety disorders are a heterogeneous group of syndromes characterized most broadly by subjective fearfulness and autonomic arousal. The protean manifestations of these disorders is reflected in the long list of signs and symptoms that may be associated (Table 7.1).

It has been relatively recently that acute episodic anxiety disorders (''panic

**Table 7.1**
Signs and Symptoms Associated with Anxiety

| Subjective | Objective |
|---|---|
| Panic | Hyperventilation |
| Feelings of unreality | Tachycardia |
| Feelings of depersonalization | Tachypnea |
| Fear of losing control | Diaphoresis |
| Dizziness | Pallor |
| Palpitations | Near-syncope |
| Irritability | Arrhythmia |
| Apprehension | Diarrhea |
| Impatience | |
| Vigilance | |
| Fatigue | |
| Insomnia | |
| Muscle tension | |
| Abdominal discomfort | |

attacks'') have been distinguished diagnostically from the more chronic anxiety disorders. There is emerging evidence that panic attacks may differ from the more chronic or generalized disorders in several ways. They may be more strongly genetically based, and the underlying neurophysiology may differ. Psychopharmacologic responsiveness differs in the syndromes (Shader *et al.*, 1982). Agoraphobia commonly coexists with panic disorders, but the relations between the anxiety disorders and other phobic conditions are less well understood. In general, it seems fair to say that our neurologic understanding of the anxiety disorders is at a more primitive level than for the other syndromes discussed in this book.

These disorders are common. Point prevalence studies in the United States indicate rates ranging from 2% to 4.7% (Shader, 1984). Although some of the prevalence studies have been flawed by imprecise diagnostic criteria, more recent studies indicate that the generalized, more chronic form of anxiety disorder accounts for 50% or more of the cases, with panic disorders and phobic disorders occurring less commonly (Weissman *et al.*, 1978). In most of these epidemiologic studies, there has been a significant preponderance of young adult women among the patients.

There are reviews in the psychosomatic literature contending that 10–40% of patients who experience anxiety disorders are experiencing, in part, an emotional manifestation of a physical illness, as opposed to a ''pure'' emotional illness (Schuckit, 1983). These rates seem high to us. Still, there is no doubt that for a number of medical and neurologic conditions, signs and symptoms of anxiety may be part of the physiology of the illness. Table 7.2 lists the more common of these conditions organized according to whether generalized or episodic anxiety is more likely to be mimicked.

One should consider that the medical evaluation of patients with generalized anxiety disorders differs somewhat from those with episodic anxiety disorders (panic attacks). Drug withdrawal syndromes are more likely to appear within the former group, whereas episodic drug dosing such as in cocaine or caffeine abuse is more likely in the latter group. Endocrine disorders may appear in either group. Most of the cardiovascular syndromes are episodic in causing symptoms, but metabolic disturbances are typically continuous. Clinicians cannot rely inflexibly on such dichotomies, of course, since considerable overlap and ambiguity may be present in the various clinical presentations of both the medical disorders and the anxiety disorders themselves.

In the evaluation of anxious patients, clinicians face not only this intrinsic overlap with several medical disorders but also the recently identified association between anxiety disorders and the affective disorders. That is, patients who

**Table 7.2**
Medical and Neurologic Syndromes Associated with Anxiety

| | Generalized | Episodic |
|---|---|---|
| Drug and toxin | Hypnotic/sedative withdrawal | Caffeinism |
| | Nicotine withdrawal | Methyl xanthine use/abuse |
| | Indomethacin | Adrenergic agonists |
| | Tricyclic antidepressant withdrawal | Dopamine agonists |
| | Cycloserine | Cocaine |
| | Antipsychotic withdrawal | Metrizamide |
| | Baclofen | Oxymetazoline |
| | Isocarboxazid | Phencyclidine |
| | Akathisia (antipsychotic-induced) | Organic solvent inhalation |
| | Anticholinergics | |
| | Lidocaine | |
| Endocrine | Hyperthyroidism | Pheochromocytoma |
| | Hypoparathyroidism | Hypoglycemia |
| | Cushing's syndrome | Hyperthyroidism |
| | Addison's disease | |
| Cardiovascular | | Mitral valve prolapse |
| | | Arrhythmia |
| | | Angina pectoris |
| Pulmonary | Chronic obstructive pulmonary disease | Pulmonary embolus |
| Metabolic | Hypoxia | Porphyria |
| | Electrolyte disturbance | |
| | Hypocalcemia | |
| Epilepsy | | Partial complex seizures |

are anxious are often depressed, and vice versa. Breier and colleagues (1984) have recently reported that 68% of patients with agoraphobia/panic disorder have a history of major depressive episodes, often occurring in juxtaposition to the anxious symptoms. Family studies have recently appeared that may indicate a genetic basis for mixed anxious/depressive syndromes, at least in some persons (Leckman *et al.*, 1983). We have no systematic knowledge concerning patterns of admixed depression among the anxiety disorders of medical and neurologic disease.

## DRUG- OR TOXIN-INDUCED ANXIETY

A 50-year-old successful businessman complained of chronic feelings of "tension," "worry," and "uptightness." On some occasions, he felt terrified and frightened quite suddenly, as if he were "fainting out" or "running out of air." When questioned about medication and drug usage during the eliciting of the past medical history, he described drinking from 6 to 12 cups of brewed coffee during the work week, when the "fainting" spells were most likely to occur.

A wide array of drugs have been reported in association with anxietylike side effects (for a review see Medical Letter, 1986). In general, however, there are two broad categories of drugs clinicians should consider during the evaluation of anxious patients. The first includes those drugs that act as direct or indirect adrenergic agonists and the phosphodiesterase inhibitors, such as caffeine, which work at the "second messenger" step beyond the adrenergic receptors. The second broad category include the early or mild withdrawal syndromes that are associated with sedatives and hypnotics.

The adrenergic agonists tend to be prescribed for patients with colds, asthma, parkinsonian diseases, narcolepsy, and hyperactivity syndromes. Many are over-the-counter preparations that contain ephedrine, pseudoephedrine, and congeners. Caffeine has properties similar to these drugs and has been associated by Greden and colleagues with reversible anxiety disorders when used in excess (Greden, 1974; Greden *et al.*, 1978). Pharmacologic effects of caffeine are not likely to occur until a dosage of 500–600 mg/day has been exceeded. Dosage estimates for some common preparations are provided in Table 7.3 (Dietch, 1981).

Cocaine is another drug with adrenergic agonist properties, which is becoming one of the most frequent drugs of abuse among young adults. There are preliminary reports of patients who experienced onset of panic disorder while snorting cocaine (Aronson and Craig, 1986). This association may be considerably more extensive, however, and it seems prudent to consider a clinical history of cocaine abuse in initial evaluations of anxious patients.

It might be remarked here that many of the adrenergic agonist sorts of

**Table 7.3**
Caffeine Content of Common Preparations

| | |
|---|---|
| OTC analgesics | 30–60 mg caffeine per tablet |
| Brewed coffee (5 oz) | 90–120 mg caffeine per cup |
| Instant coffee (5 oz) | 70 mg caffeine |
| Tea (5 oz) | 70 mg caffeine |
| Cola drinks (5 oz) | 20 mg caffeine |

drugs we have listed here were also listed in the previous chapter, "Manic Syndrome." This is true, but the explanation of it is far from clear. What is it that determines one person's hypomanic response to a drug such as amantadine, whereas another person becomes anxious? We do not know. There is some evidence that anxiety disorders are associated with alterations within those central neurotransmitter systems that have been most closely linked with the affective disorders, namely serotonin and norepinephrine (Hoehn-Saric, 1982). Such evidence might help us to understand the common list of drugs associated with the two clinical syndromes, but not the differential clinical responses. These are areas for future research.

By far the most common drug-induced anxiety disorder is that associated with early or partial withdrawal from sedative hypnotic drugs, especially alcohol. Occult abusers of such drugs who develop anxiety symptoms are more difficult to recognize than known abusers, and this may partly explain the prevalence of benzodiazepine and similar prescriptions which are written for alcoholics. Emergence of early withdrawal syndromes in such occult abusers is likely to occur in settings that diminish their access to drug supplies. Signs and symptoms of an anxiety disorder that emerge 1–2 days after admission to the hospital, for example, are suspicious for a withdrawal syndrome. Over 30 years ago, May and other writers reported that the entire spectrum of clinical psychiatry may be mimicked or caricatured by withdrawal syndromes (May and Ebaugh, 1953). In our experience, however, generalized anxiety disorder is most easily confused with withdrawal, since even certain physical findings are common to both clinical situations. The appearance of the withdrawal syndrome is a function of several factors, including the half-life of the addictive drug, the severity of the addiction in terms of amount consumed per 24 hr, and others. The signs and symptoms of withdrawal may appear after one or two half-lives have elapsed. Half-lives for some representative sedative drugs and routes of metabolism are presented in Table 7.4. Chronic partial withdrawal states may be encountered that persist for periods of weeks and months.

Withdrawal from beta-blocking medications may also produce signs and symptoms of generalized anxiety, but this appears to be much less frequent than other withdrawal states (Williams *et al.*, 1979).

**Table 7.4**
Elimination Half-Lives of Sedative Hypnotic Drugs

| Drug | Half-life | Principal metabolism |
|---|---|---|
| Ethanol | 18–25 mg hr | Hepatic oxidation–zero order kinetics |
| Diazepam (Valium) | 24–48 hr | Hepatic glucuronide conjugation |
| Chlordiazepoxide (Librium) | 24–48 hr | Hepatic glucuronide conjugation |
| Lorazepam | 12 hr | Hepatic glucuronide conjugation |
| Oxazepam | 10–14 hr | Hepatic glucuronide conjugation |
| Pentobarbital | 15–50 hr | Hepatic microsomal metabolism |

## Demographics

Alcoholism is probably more common than any other medical disorder profiled in this book. It is probably discussed less often than most of these other disorders (i.e., TWUD factor is less than 1*). Perhaps 10 million Americans suffer from the illness. Men appear to become alcoholic at a higher rate than women, but all ages, races, and social classes are affected. The prudent approach for the clinician is to "bracket" any demographic stereotypes that he or she may carry and to consider all adults at risk for alcoholism. Incidence and prevalence data for caffeinism and other forms of sedative hypnotic abuse are not so well known.

## Clinical History

Caffeine consumption is usually elicited by the interviewer in a straightforward manner. The same is often true for sedative hypnotic drugs, at least when they are physician-prescribed. The clinical history of alcohol consumption is a more emotionally charged area, in which reliable historical data must often come from an observer other than the patient. This is one of those rare situations in which the physical and laboratory examination may speak louder than the clinical history.

## Psychotropic Drug Interaction

None are specific to sedative hypnotic or psychostimulant usage.

*The TWUD factor is an acronym from academic medicine referring to "time wasted in useless discussion." It is the ratio of times a disease or condition is discussed on rounds to the number of times it is actually encountered.

## Mental Status Examination

Useful reports of cognitive alterations during psychostimulant-induced anxiety states are not available. In the withdrawal states, especially those related to alcohol, tests that assess *attention* and *concentration* are most useful: serial digit repetition; serial subtraction; alternating M/N test. Impairments on these tests are useful for following the patient's clinical course as well.

## General Medical Examination

Our observations here apply primarily to alcohol abuse and alcohol withdrawal anxiety.

Vital Signs. Remember that during withdrawal, patients who are dependent on sedative–hypnotic drugs may develop volume depletion, cardiac arrhythmias, and autonomic instability. Observe actively for fever, tachycardia, cardiac arrhythmia, and postural hypotension (systolic BP decrement of 20 mm Hg or more as patient moves from supine to erect position). (Alcohol intoxication itself may induce arrhythmias.)

HEENT. Facial flushing; rhinophyma.

GI. Hepatomegaly; stool guaiac for occult blood. Alcoholics typically have small, cirrhotic livers, although hepatomegaly may be present during episodes of acute alcoholic hepatitis. The liver should not exceed 10–12 cm in the midclavicular line by palpation or percussion. Hepatomegaly may also indicate cancer.

Skin. Spider angiomata; icterus.

## Neurological Examination

Cranial Nerves. Persistent *nystagmus* on lateral gaze should not be seen in the "psychiatric" anxiety syndromes. *Disconjugate gaze* may be seen in serious or advanced alcoholic disorders (i.e., Wernicke-Korsakoff syndrome).

Sensory. Is there evidence of peripheral neuropathy? Findings commonly include stocking/glove pattern of impaired sensitivity to pin or touch, absent ankle reflexes, and painful dysesthesias across plantar surfaces of feet. Few people like the Babinski maneuver, but alcoholics like it even less.

Motor. Postural tremor, distal > proximal, may be present in early withdrawal. Evidence of cerebellar impairment may be present in chronic abusers of alcohol, especially midline or vermian cerebellar impairment. Patients should be checked for ability to perform the Romberg maneuver and to perform the tandem walk. Abnormalities on these tests may prove transient in some cases, related to the withdrawal state.

Reflexes. May be hyperactive in withdrawal but should be symmetric. Babinski signs are not acceptable as part of mild or early withdrawal states. Remember that drug abusers (especially alcohol abusers) are at greater risk for head injury than other patients and possibly are at greater risk for stroke.

## Laboratory and Imaging

A *blood alcohol level* is often present during early withdrawal. Some general relationships between blood alcohol levels and degrees of clinical intoxication are provided in Table 7.5 (Miles, 1922). The correlations presented in Table 7.5 are derived from nonaddicted subjects and may not apply well to persons with high or chronic alcohol consumption, who can tolerate considerably higher serum levels of the drug.

SMA-6. Serum electrolytres, BUN, and glucose should be checked for evidence of hypernatremia, hyponatremia, hypokalemia, and hyper- and hypoglycemia. The anion gap may be increased in alcohol abusers owing to the presence of unmeasured anions such as lactate, pyruvate, B-hydroxybutyrate, and acetoacetate (Goldfrank and Starke, 1979).

$$\text{Anion gap} = (Na^+ + K^+) - (HCO_3^- + C1^-) \qquad \text{(normal is 12–16)}$$

If the anion gap is increased, arterial blood gases should be checked to confirm a pattern of metabolic acidosis.

**Table 7.5**
Relationships between Blood Alcohol and Clinical State

| Blood alcohol | Clinical features |
|---|---|
| 30 mg/dl (0.03%) | Mild euphoria |
| 50 mg/dl (0.05%) | Mild incoordination |
| 100 mg/dl (0.10%) | Ataxia |
| 200 mg/dl (0.20%) | Arousal impairments |
| 300 mg/dl (0.30%) | Stupor |
| 400 mg/dl (0.40%) | Anesthesia/coma |

SMA-12. Elevated liver enzymes—ALT, AST, ALK phosphatase LDH.

CBC. Macrocytosis.

## ENDOCRINE-INDUCED ANXIETY DISORDERS

A 58-year-old woman was referred from OB GYN to psychiatry for treatment of a generalized anxiety disorder. For a year or two she had felt increasingly nervous, fidgety, and apprehensive. She perspired easily under stress and now slept fitfully. The gynecologist had prescribed benzodiazepines with some initial benefit, but the woman's complaints had recurred. Upon first contact with the woman, the psychiatrist noticed bilateral widening of the palpebral fissures.

There are several endocrine disorders that have been associated with anxiety symptoms (Table 7.2). The evidence for an association with hyperthyroidism seems strongest, and we will discuss this particular endocrine disorder in some detail. Pheochromocytoma is a rare disorder but should also be considered within this group of psychiatric disorders. Cushing's disease is discussed in Chapter 5, since it is more commonly associated with torpor and depressivelike symptoms. Hypoparathyroidism, hypoglycemia, disorders of calcium, and Addison's disease are profiled more briefly.

### Hyperthyroidism

Hyperthyroid patients sometimes develop psychosis, dementia, or affective disorders. They *commonly* develop signs and symptoms that are akin to the anxiety disorders. This is not surprising when one considers that the clinical signs and symptoms that correlate best with hyperthyroidism include palpitations, fatigue, preference for cold, diaphoresis, nervousness, increased appetite, weight loss, thyroid enlargement, hyperkinetic movements, tachycardia, and atrial fibrillation (Crooks *et al.*, 1959). In series of consecutive patients with clinical hyperthyroidism of various causes, one can expect that two-thirds or more will meet DSM-III criteria for an anxiety disorder (Kathol *et al.*, 1986). Our evidence for this association moving "in the other direction" from screening studies of anxiety/panic patients for thyroid disease is more tentative (Stein, 1986). There is some evidence that panic disorder patients demonstrate higher than expected rates of thyroid disease by clinical history, but laboratory confirmation has not been definitive.

Fortunately or unfortunately for psychiatrists, both hyperthyroidism and many of the anxiety disorders are diseases of women in early-adult and middle-adult life (Chopra and Solomon, 1983). The causes of thyrotoxic states are presented in Table 7.6. The diseases in group I are associated with intrinsic

**Table 7.6**
Diseases That Produce Thyrotoxicosis

| Group I | Group II |
|---|---|
| TSH-producing adenoma | Thyrotoxicosis factitia |
| Graves' disease | Subacute thyroiditis |
| Hyperfunctioning adenoma | Chronic thyroiditis |
| Toxic multinodular goiter | Trophoblastic tumor |
| | Struma ovarii |

hyperfunction of the thyroid gland and typically are associated with an increased radioactive iodine uptake (RAIU), whereas those in group II usually demonstrate a decreased RAIU.

Graves' disease is by far the most common of the diseases in group I. Graves' disease is an autoimmune disease characterized by the clinical signs of toxic goiter, ophthalmopathy, and dermopathy. All three of the clinical features may not be present. Familial clustering and genetic predisposition occur in the disease. The pathophysiology is not fully understood, but it has to do with the action of an immune-related extrinsic thyroid-stimulating material that circulates in the plasma. Occasionally other autoimmune phenomena are associated, such as vitiligo or pernicious anemia.

Hashimoto's thyroiditis is the most common of the diseases in group II. It, too, is an autoimmune thyroid disease which favors women over men, but it tends to occur through a middle-life age range as opposed to the earlier onset of Graves' disease. In Hashimoto's thyroiditis an inflammatory infiltrate of the thyroid occurs, producing goiter, and eventually hypothyroidism due to fibrous replacement of the gland. Hyperthyroidism may appear early in the disease course, perhaps owing to a common association of this syndrome with Graves' disease (Hamburger, 1986).

In people over 60 years of age, hyperthyroidism may still occur, but it is more commonly due to toxic nodular goiter than to Graves' disease (Hurley, 1983). The onset of the hyperthyroid state may be more insidious in this condition than in the thyrotoxic syndromes of earlier life. Moreover, many of the clinical signs and symptoms detailed below may not be present. "Apathetic" as opposed to "anxious" hyperthyroidism, for example, is a behavioral syndrome of the elderly.

Before describing the clinical and laboratory profiles of thyrotoxicosis, we remind the reader that this background discussion of thyroid disease is extremely global and brief. It will substitute poorly for a good textbook of internal medicine.

## Demographics

For the autoimmune hyperthyroid conditions (Graves' disease; Hashimoto's thyroiditis), women outnumber men 6:1. This ratio decreases in toxic multinodular goiter and approaches parity for the hyperthyroid states of late life.

## Clinical History

There are a number of historical clues that can alert the clinician with the possibility of intercurrent endocrine disease in a patient with generalized anxiety disorder or panic disorder:

**Family History.** Patients with thyroid disease typically have a family history positive for thyroid disease, especially among female relations. Patients with anxiety disorders may well have a family history positive for anxiety disorders. One should take notice when such family histories are reversed.

**Past Medical History.** One should ask specifically concerning associated autoimmune diseases, such as megaloblastic anemia, myasthenia gravis, and systemic lupus erythematosus.

**Past Psychiatric History.** A clinical clue we have found useful is that hyperthyroid/anxious patients typically have no premorbid history of psychopathology or of psychological dysfunction. Anxious patients, on the other hand, will commonly state that they were "always on the nervous side," even if the overt disorders did not begin until a later time in their lives.

### Review of Systems Clues

*HEENT*. Dysphagia?

*Respiratory*. Dyspnea?

*Cardiac*. Palpitations? Atrial fibrillation? Congestive heart failure? Exacerbation of angina? All of those complaints are of greater note when offered spontaneously by the patient.

*GI*. Diarrhea?

*Endocrine*. Weight loss? Heat intolerance? Diaphoresis?

## Psychotropic Drug Interactions

There is a series of case reports to suggest that hyperthyroidism enhances susceptibility to severe extrapyramidal side effects of antipsychotic drugs (Witschy and Redmond, 1981). There are other reports to suggest that an idiosyncratic reaction to antipsychotics may occur in such patients, characterized by fever, tachycardia, diaphoresis, and even sudden death (Hoffman *et al.*, 1978; Weiner, 1979). Most of these reports implicate the high-potency drugs, such as haloperidol. At this point, it may be prudent to avoid such high-potency antipsychotics in patients with known or suspected hyperthyroidism.

Lithium also interacts with thyroid metabolism (Wilson and Jefferson, 1985). Clinical or laboratory evidence of hypothyroidism may appear in 5–30% of patients on lithium maintenance, although this is usually reversible upon withdrawal of the drug.

Carbamazepine has also been the subject of several reports associating it with decreases in serum $T_4$ and $T_3$. The clinical significance of this is not yet known.

## Mental Status Examination

Anecdotal reports indicate a quality of irritability and fatigue occurring in the anxiety syndrome associated with hyperthyroidism, but such observations are of little diagnostic utility. In one report it seemed clear that cognitive disturbances were *not* part of the hyperthyroid clinical picture (Heinik, 1986).

## General Medical Examination

HEENT. Hair—fine and silken? Thyromegaly? Reptilian stare with infrequent blinking? Lid lag? Proptosis, unilateral or bilateral? Careful observation of head and neck during the interview is prudent in evaluating anxious patients.

Cardiac. Tachycardia? Atrial fibrillation? Widened pulse pressure?

Skin. Warm or diaphoretic? Localized pretibial myxedema may be seen in Graves' disease; a circumscribed, thickened or pigmented area across the tibial surface. Nails—onycholysis.

## Neurological Examination

Cranial Nerves. Exophthalmos? Extraocular muscle limitations? This may be the time to pay explicit attention to orbital and periorbital structures.

Sensory. Not remarkable.

Motor. Fine tremor may be seen, usually postural with wrists extended. Weakness may be seen in hyperthyroid patients but should not be present in anxious patients or in *hypo*thyroid patients. All three groups may complain of weakness, but only in the hyperthyroid patients should it prove objective. Occasionally, there is proximal wasting of hip and shoulder girdle musculature in such patients.

Reflexes. Diffuse hyperreflexia is not invariable, but it is usually present in those patients who have the fine postural tremor.

### Laboratory and Imaging

Sophisticated endocrine testing for hyperthyroidism quickly becomes a matter for subspecialists. We here provide an overview and conceptual framework which we hope will facilitate initial evaluations and more effective consultation. Several principles should be borne in mind. One is that serum $T_4$ is reversibly bound to thyroxine-binding globulin (TBG) and medical conditions that may increase TBG may produce an artifactual elevation in $T_4$. Pregnancy, liver disease, estrogen therapy, and narcotic drug abuse are several such conditions. Tests that "get around" this difficulty and produce an index of free or unbound thyroid hormones include the $T_3$ resin uptake and the free thyroxine index. The $T_3$ resin uptake measures the number of unoccupied $T_4$ binding sites in serum. Thus, it is elevated in true hyperthyroidism and decreased in hypothyroidism. The free $T_4$ index is calculated from the $T_4$ and $T_3$ resin uptake. Normal values for serum thyroid tests are as follows (New England Journal of Medicine, 1986):

| | |
|---|---|
| Thyroid-stimulating hormone (TSH) | 0.5–5.0 $\mu$U/ml |
| Thyroxine-binding globulin capacity | 15–25 $\mu$g $T_4$/100 ml |
| Total triiodothyronine ($T_3$) | 75–195 ng/100ml |
| Reverse triiodothyronine ($rT_3$) | 13–53 ng/ml |
| Total thyroxine by RIA ($T_4$) | 4–12 $\mu$g/100ml |
| $T_3$ resin uptake | 25–35% |
| Free thyroxine index ($FT_4I$) | 1–4 |

An outline approach to the laboratory evaluation of patients suspected of having hyperthyroidism is presented in Fig. 7.1.

## Pheochromocytoma

Pheochromocytoma may be looked for more often, and found less often, than any other medical disease. Wilson's disease and porphyria (also discussed in this chapter) probably run close seconds. Although we may make fun of ourselves for occasionally "chasing" these relatively rare diseases, we must

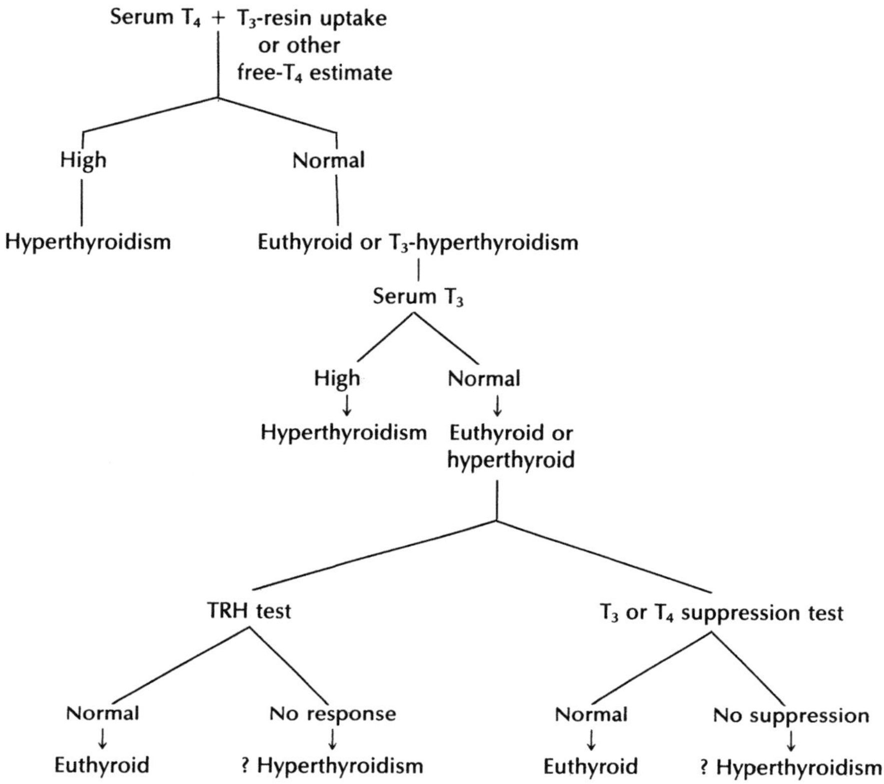


**Figure 7.1.** Laboratory approach to hyperthyroidism. (From Kaplan and Utiger, 1978. Reprinted with permission.)

remind ourselves that this sort of chase *is* the physician's responsibility. It is not funny when psychiatric patients are harmed by undiagnosed and treatable medical illness.

Pheochromocytomas are abdominal tumors of young to middle-adult life which present with catecholamine-mediated "crises." Since some of the anxiety disorders are, in a sense, catecholamine-mediated crises as well, psychiatrists should have some familiarity with these catecholamine-secreting tumors. The tumors typically secrete a mixture of epinephrine and norepinephrine, and the clinical attacks result from sudden rises in serum levels of these hormones. Typical symptoms and signs include facial flushing, headache, vertigo, hypertension, tachycardia, diaphoresis, dyspnea, chest pain, tremor, and nausea. When a series of patients with active pheochromocytomas were compared with anxiety disorder patients, symptoms of headache and diaphoresis occurred much more frequently among the pheochromocytoma patients (Starkman *et al.*, 1985). Persistent hypertension was present in the majority of these patients as well.

The clinical picture that should turn the clinician's attention to this diagnostic possibility is an anxiety disorder associated with hypertension, headache, or diaphoresis.

## Demographics

These tumors are abdominal chromaffin cell tumors of young to middle-adult life. There may be a slight female preponderance, and occasionally there is familial clustering.

## Clinical History

One should listen for a history of discrete episodes or "crises" that are clearly *not* related to emotional events, especially if complaints of headache and sweating are intermingled. Of course, this history does not necessarily distinguish such crises from panic attacks. In Starkman's report the panic disorder patients were more likely than the pheochromocytoma patients to complain of fear of dying, fears of freeze attacks, and unsteady walking.

## Psychotropic Drug Interactions

**Tricyclic Antidepressants.** By blocking catecholamine reuptake mechanisms, these drugs may produce sudden, serious exacerbation of crises or hypertension. They should not be used when a clinical suspicion of pheochromocytoma is present. These drugs also interfere with laboratory testing for catecholamines and their metabolites.

**Monoamine Oxidase Inhibitors.** These drugs may decrease excretion of vanillylmandelic acid (VMA), interfering with diagnostic laboratory testing (see below). They artifactually *increase* metanephrine excretion. They too are potentially dangerous in pheochromocytoma patients.

**Chlorpromazine.** May also falsely elevate urinary assays for catechole metabolites (Dietch, 1981).

## Mental Status Examination

Aside from symptomatic differences earlier described, no distinguishing features have been reported.

### General Medical Examination

Vital Signs. Hypertension; tachycardia, sometimes occurring between crises as well as during them.

GI. The tumors are usually small and unilateral in a suprarenal location. On occasion, a large one may be palpable. After deep palpation in paravertebral areas, one can recheck blood pressure and heart rate for evidence of a sudden surge secondary to catecholamines released by the palpation.

### Neurological Examination

Findings other than postural tremor related to catecholamine surges have not been reported.

### Laboratory and Imaging

The key diagnostic tests include urinary assays for three substances: unconjugated or "free" catecholamines, vanillylmandelic acid, and metanephrines. Normal limits for 24-hr urinary excretion of these substances are provided in Table 7.7 (Bravo *et al.*, 1979). When a catecholamine-secreting tumor is present, these normal limits are usually exceeded by severalfold, as opposed to a marginal excess of either the parent compound or a metabolite. Excretion may also be falsely normal if a recent crisis has not occurred. The interference of psychotropic drugs with these test values must be kept in mind.

## Hypoglycemia

"Low blood sugar" ranks with "tired blood" and constipation as major health threats in the collective preconscious of Western civilization. In fact, true hypoglycemia is quite rare. Glucose is the major metabolic substrate for

**Table 7.7**
Normal 24-hr Urine Excretions for Catecholamines and Metabolites

| | Upper limit |
|---|---|
| Epinephrine | 50 $\mu$g |
| Norepinephrine | 100 $\mu$g |
| Metanephrine | 1.3 mg |
| VMA | 7.0 mg |

the brain, and several endocrine systems are in place to maintain serum glucose. When true hypoglycemia does occur, however, it may produce symptoms reminiscent of anxiety. People may feel tremulous, hyperalert, diaphoretic, apprehensive, and hungry. These symptoms tend to appear when the glucose is in the range of 30–45 mg%. If the level reaches 30 mg% and lower, a stuporous and lethargic condition may supervene. There is very little evidence that true hypoglycemia occurs with any frequency among anxious/panic patients (Stein, 1986).

In general, there are three conditions in which symptomatic hypoglycemia may be seen. One is drug-induced (insulin, and the oral hypoglycemic agents); a second is insulinoma-induced hypoglycemia; and a third is "reactive" hypoglycemia. This last group includes the transient hypoglycemic states that may be associated with gastrectomy or short bowel syndromes and occasionally endocrine disorders such as prediabetes or hypothyroidism. The reactive hypoglycemias may sometimes be identified by performing a glucose tolerance test and documenting symptoms associated with a serum glucose below 45 mg% (Levine, 1974). A serum glucose during an anxiety attack itself is best. It is very important to document a true association between the low glucose and the clinical symptoms under investigation.

### Clinical History

Reactive hypoglycemia may occur in a regular pattern around meals—i.e., symptoms always 1 hr after lunch. A history of bowel surgery may also raise clinical suspicion. Without the presence of one of these factors in the clinical situation, the likelihood of finding hypoglycemia is so low as to obviate the need for further investigation.

### Laboratory and Imaging

Three-hour glucose challenge for reactive hypoglycemia: Oral load of 75 g glucose, followed by serum glucose determinations at 30, 60, 90, 120, and 180. No value should be less than 45 mg%, and symptoms should be noted. Some patients who are observed through 4 or 5 hr may demonstrate serum glucoses in the range of 40–45 mg%, but this is of questionable significance.

## Hypoparathyroidism

A majority of patients with hypoparathyroidism demonstrate mental status changes, probably secondary to decreased serum calcium. In Denko and Kaebling's 1962 review of the literature prior to 1962, they concluded that diffuse cognitive deterioration was the most common alteration of mental status seen in such patients. A substantial minority are described with prominant emotional findings, however, including nervousness, irritability, hypochondriosis, and panic attacks. Muscular irritability and spontaneous fractures are also seen. The universe of patients at risk for this phenomenon is not large—primarily those who have undergone neck dissections for thyroid or parathyroid disease or cancer. Hypoparathyroidism may also occur on an idiopathic basis, and low serum calcium may be induced by unusual diets and by malignancy (Carlson, 1986).

## Clinical History

Has the patient had neck surgery? The onset of clinically significant hypoparathyroidism usually occurs several days after the surgery, but it may continue for months if unrecognized. Is there a history of unusual diet, which might be low in calcium? Is there a reason to suspect malignancy, particularly one capable of taking up calcium, such as prostatic carcinoma?

## General Medical Examination

**Chvostek's Sign.** A tap of the proximal facial nerve produces ipsilateral contraction of muscles such as buccinator, frontalis, and orbicularis. This sign is a manifestation of tetany.

**Trousseau's Sign.** Trousseau's sign refers to carpopedal spasm following application of blood pressure cuff and inflation to systolic pressure in a limb.

**Hyperventilation.** Simple hyperventilation by temporarily reducing the amount of ionized calcium available may also precipitate carpopedal spasm. Unfortunately, some simply anxious patients are able to accomplish this after hyperventilation, so the sign is not conclusive per se.

## Laboratory and Imaging

| | Normal ranges |
|---|---|
| Serum hypocalcemia | 8.5–10.5 mg/100 ml (2.20–2.58 mmole/liter) |
| Hyperphosphatemia | 3.0–4.5 mg/100 ml (0.32–1.40 mmole/liter) |
| Normal renal function | Creatinine 0.6–1.5 mg/100 ml (50–110 mmole/liter) |
| Low or absent serum parathyroid hormone | |
| Ionized calcium | 2.00–2.30 meq/liter (1.00–1.15 mmole/liter) |

It should be remembered that abnormalities of liver function, albumin levels, and renal function may alter individual values for calcium or phosphorus. Ionized calcium determination may be more reliable under such circumstances.

## CARDIOVASCULAR-INDUCED ANXIETY DISORDERS

Do patients with acute and chronic anxiety disorders have an increased prevalence of mitral valve prolapse? And if they do, are there any treatment implications of this cardiac abnormality that should be considered by psychiatrists? We frame these issues in the form of two questions, since our present state of research does not admit definite answers to either.

Mitral valve prolapse (MVP) refers to the herniation of mitral leaflets backward into the left atrium during systole. This functional cardiac abnormality may be quite common among young women, who may have prevalence rates in the range of 10%. The finding seems to be less common among men and older women. Typical physical findings include an early or midsystolic click heard best along the left sternal border, which may be followed by a soft systolic murmur. There is some evidence that a particular body habitus may be associated with MVP; straight back, tall and lean build, with pectus excavatum or a narrow anteroposterior chest diameter (Rosenman, 1985).

There is disagreement in the psychiatric literature concerning a possible association between MVP and chronic anxiety or panic (Bowen *et al.*, 1985; Szmuilowicz and Flannery, 1980). When series of patients with anxiety disorders (especially panic disorder) are examined for MVP by clinical examination or two-dimensional echocardiogram, it appears that 30–50% demonstrate prolapse (Liberthson *et al.*, 1986; Maturzas *et al.*, 1987). Similarly, when series of patients with MVP established by examination and echocardiogram are assessed for anxiety symptoms, they appear more "anxious" than normal controls (Mazza *et al.*, 1986). What is unclear in many of these reports is whether subtle selection biases have entered into the case-finding process. In addition, the reliability of the echocardiograph determinations has been questioned (Gorman *et al.*, 1986). On balance, it seems reasonable to conclude at the present time that patients with anxiety/panic disorders *do* have a greater frequency of mitral valve abnormalities than do controls, but the clinical significance of this remains unclear.

An equally difficult question is whether patients with MVP need medical treatment, such as aspirin anticoagulation, for their valvular disease. The best answer to this seems to be that all prolapses are not equal in terms of pathophysiology and prognosis (Wynne, 1986). There is evidence that those patients with MVP who are at risk for progressive valvular incompetence, stroke, and arrhythmia are those who have thickening of the valve beyond 5 mm in addi-

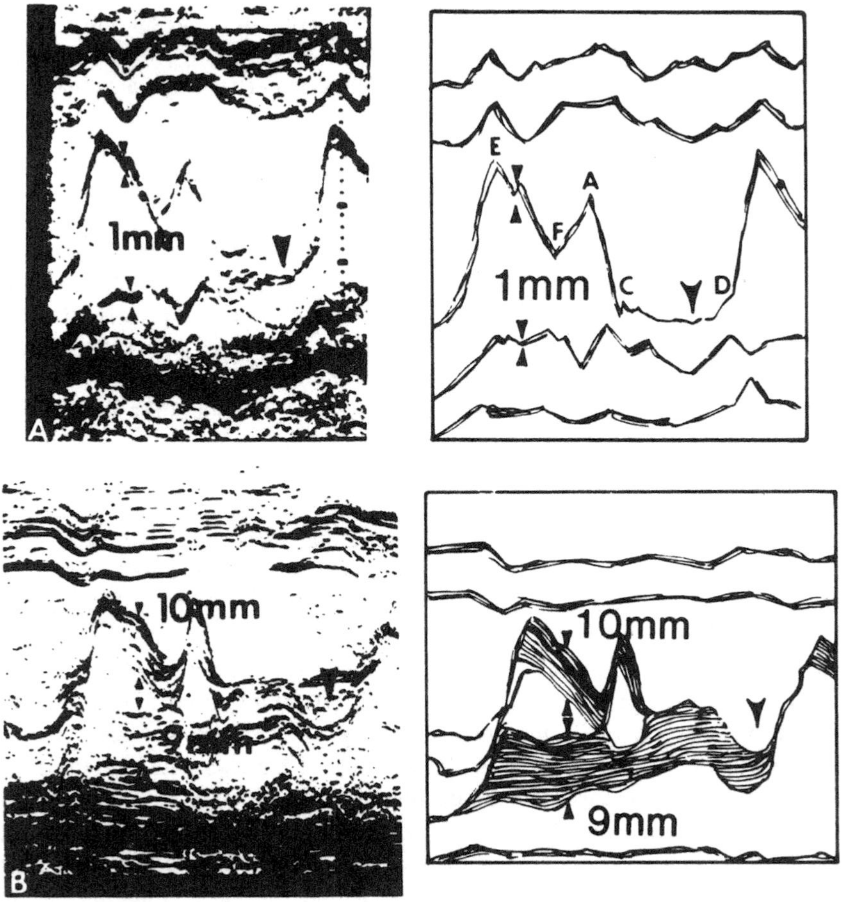


**Figure 7.2.** M-Mode echocardiographic recordings (left) and artist's representation of mitral valve (right), demonstrating method of measuring "thickness" of mitral valve leaflet (see text). Large arrowheads indicate systolic prolapse. Small arrowheads indicate measurements of leaflet thickness. Panel A shows the normal thickness of anterior and posterior leaflets; panel B, the increased thickness of anterior and posterior leaflets. The letters A, C, D, E, and F denote various points on the M-mode mitral valve echocardiogram (see text).

tion to the prolapse (Nishimura *et al.*, 1985). Figure 7.2 presents typical echocardiographic configurations of prolapse with normal valvular leaflets, and prolapse with thickened leaflets.

Two other cardiovascular disorders that have been reported in association with anxietylike symptoms include angina pectoris and various cardiac arrhythmias. In our experience, these processes are not easily confounded. Although patients who become suddenly hypotensive from an arrhythmia or who develop angina may have some symptoms resembling anxiety, the remainder of the clinical context is usually quite distinctive. Moreover, the age ranges tend to be disparate, with anxiety disorders beginning early in adult life and the cardiac diseases later.

## Demographics

For some reason, mitral valve prolapse seems to be diagnosed much more commonly among women in their 20s (prevalence rates of perhaps 17%) than among women in their 60s, when prevalence rates fall to approximately 5% (Savage *et al.*, 1983). Men receive the diagnosis at a much lower rate.

## Clinical History

Our present feeling is that the "benign" form of MVP (i.e., prolapse without thickening of the leaflets) is clinically indistinguishable from anxiety disorders *without* valvular abnormalities. In taking the history, therefore, one seeks to elicit evidence that none of the more worrisome sorts of valvular or other cardiac disease might be present. For example:

Cardiac. A history of rheumatic heart disease, infarction, or arrhythmia would be of concern. Many patients with panic attacks feel their heart "pounding" during the attack, or "racing," but they do not usually say that it is irregular. Chest pain itself should not be part of the clinical picture.

Neurologic. Although many anxious patients feel lightheaded during symptomatic periods, and some will actually describe dramatic swooning or slumping events, true loss of consciousness is unusual.

## Psychotropic Drug Interactions

Three categories of psychotropic drugs are generally prescribed for the various anxiety disorders: benzodiazepines, tricyclic antidepressants, and monoamine oxidase inhibitors. There is no specific interaction with the cardiac syndromes described above, except for the prolongation of intracardiac conduction, which may be induced by the tricyclics.

## Mental Status Examination

The mental status findings in the various anxiety conditions associated with valvular heart disease have not been reported to differ from those in other anxiety disorders.

## General Medical Examination

*Cardiac*: (1) Rhythm, (2) systolic clicks especially early in systole, and (3) systolic murmurs, which may be louder in expiration, as ventricular filling and size decrease.

## Neurological Examination

Patients with anxiety/panic disorder commonly present with somatic symptoms and concerns. Many feel more comfortable with general medical physicians and come only reluctantly to psychiatrists. We would like to say that these patients have symptoms without signs and that their neurologic examinations are normal. Unfortunately, many of them do have "focal-like" examinations and complaints, especially focal sensory findings, focal clumsiness and weakness, and blurred vision (Coyle and Sterman, 1986). These signs can be attributed to the anxiety disorder itself when they are transient and associated only with panic symptomatology or increased anxious symptoms.

## Laboratory and Imaging

Electrocardiogram. May provide clues to rhythm abnormalities. A variety of abnormalities may indicate that patients have a more serious form of valvular disease. T-wave inversions in precordial leads may occur as part of MVP.

Holter Monitor. Twelve or 24-hr studies should be performed when significant rhythm disturbance is suspected.

Echocardiogram. See Fig. 7.2. This is currently the most sensitive diagnostic test for MVP, but it may identify as "abnormal" some functional bulging of the valve, which is physiologic. It is probably most valuable when thickness of leaflets are assessed as well as prolapse.

# PULMONARY-RELATED ANXIETY DISORDERS

Hypoxia makes conscious people anxious. Jefferson and Marshall (1981) have stated that clinicians who forget this maxim leave themselves liable for one of the most embarrassing diagnostic errors: "Perhaps the greatest diagnostic pitfall lies in mistaking the restlessness and apprehension of an early hypoxic delirium for psychologically based anxiety." In actual psychiatric practice, this diagnostic issue does not often arise, because most anxiety disorders occur in young and "healthy" people, and most hypoxic conditions occur in older people with diagnosed cardiorespiratory disease. Beware of a "new" anxiety diagnosis in middle-aged people who have cardiorespiratory disease.

The list of medical disorders capable of producing hypoxia is too long for this discussion, but we would like to comment on occult pulmonary embolus. When new anxiety symptoms appear in a patient at bed rest for whatever reason, this diagnostic possibility should immediately come to mind. The chest x-ray is commonly unremarkable in this situation, and the arterial blood gases may be normal, especially if delayed until symptoms begin to improve. A good rule to follow is:

---

*Clinical Rule No. 7.1:* New anxiety disorder + bed rest = ventilation–perfusion scan + phlebogram

---

## General Medical Examination

Vital Signs. Count respirations and observe them carefully. A respiratory rate greater than 20 per minute, hyperpnea, and supraclavicular or intercostal retractions are suspicious.

Skin. Cyanosis.

Chest. Diminished breath sounds, or focal pleuritic rub over an area of embolic infarction. Any systolic or continuous murmurs across lung fields may indicate pulmonary vasculature blockade.

Musculoskeletal. Check calves and medial thigh regions carefully for erythema, swelling, palpable thrombosed veins.

## Laboratory and Imaging

EKG. Usually normal, but with embolization a right shift of axis may be seen, or tall peaked p waves.

Chest X-Ray. May show infiltrate, or infiltrate abutting the pleura if infarction has occurred.

Arterial Blood Gases. Often normal, but the pattern to be seen in pulmonary embolus often includes:

| | |
|---|---|
| Hypoxemia | $pO_2 < 70$ mm depending on age |
| Hypocapnea | $pCO_2 < 40$ mm |
| Respiratory alkalosis | $pH > 7.40$ |

Pulmonary Perfusion and Ventilation Scan. The perfusion scan is obtained by gamma camera imaging of the distribution of intravenously injected gamma-emitting radionuclides. Normal scans exhibit homogeneous distributions of radioactivity, but in embolization there may be sharply demarcated zones of diminished activity on the perfusion scan. The ventilation scan may not show concomitant decreased ventilation in these areas, thereby indicating the ventilation–perfusion mismatch which is seen early after PE.

Ascending Contrast Phlebogram. The definitive test for deep leg vein thrombosis, which is the most common origin of pulmonary emboli.

## METABOLIC-RELATED ANXIETY DISORDERS

The human organism may experience an infinite (or nearly infinite) number of possible metabolic derangements, but very few of them mimic anxiety in any serious way. We have already discussed one such syndrome, the hypoglycemia associated with hypoparathyroidism. Most of these metabolic derangements produce states of delirium, or metabolic encephalopathy. Although anxious features may be admixed, they are usually set in contrast with prominent abnormalities of arousal and concentration on the mental status examination and with motor system abnormalities on the neurologic examination.

There are two somewhat rare metabolic diseases that are occasionally associated with anxious and hysterical features—Wilson's disease and acute intermittent porphyria (AIP). We have chosen to discuss AIP in this chapter and Wilson's disease in the subsequent chapter, on nonparanoid psychoses, despite the somewhat arbitrary nature of this division.

### Acute Intermittent Porphyria

The porphyrias are a group of diseases in which there are abnormalities in the complex biosynthetic pathway of porphyrins and hemoglobin (Tschudy *et al.*, 1975; Pathak and West, 1982). We will confine our discussion to acute intermittent porphyria, since this is the one that has been reported in association with episodic and chronic neurologic and psychiatric dysfunction.

AIP is a genetically based disease of autosomal-dominant inheritance pattern, which is expressed more frequently in women than in men. Of the eight enzymatic synthetic steps in hemebiosynthesis, the enzyme that is deficient in AIP is that which catalyzes the condensation of multiple porphobilinogen molecules to form a polypyrrole, uroporphyrinogen I synthetase (now termed porphobilinogen deaminase). The more proximal rate-controlling enzyme in the sequence is delta-aminolevulinic acid synthetase, which is inducible in liver

**Table 7.8**
Risk Categories of Drugs for Precipitation of AIP

| Dangerous drugs | Safe drugs |
|---|---|
| All barbiturates | Codeine |
| All sulfonamides | Meperidine |
| All anticonvulsants except bromides, clonazapam, and possibly carbamazepine | Phenothiazines |
| | Penicillins |
| | Cephalosporins |
| Phenylbutazone | Chloramphenicol |
| Griseofulvin | Gentamycin |
| Synthetic estrogens and progestogens | Tetracyclines |
| Amphetamines | Nitrofurantoin |
| Ergot alkaloids | Mandelamine |
| | Most antihistamines |
| | Tricyclic antidepressants |
| | Antiemetics such as meclizine |
| | Corticosteroids |
| | General anesthetics |
| | Thyroid and antithyroid drugs |
| | Digitalis |
| | Vitamins A–E |
| | Diuretics |
| | Antimalarials |
| | Antihypertensive drugs |
| | Anticholinesterases |
| | Anticholinergics |

by a variety of drugs and metabolic events. When this rate-controlling enzyme is induced to a higher rate of activity, the precursor porphobilinogen molecules "back up" behind the deficient enzyme, and the clinical and biochemical manifestations of an acute attack are produced.

Four categories of events seem capable of inducing the rate-controlling enzyme and thereby the attacks; drugs, endogenous steroids related to the menstrual cycle, starvation, and infections. It is debated whether emotional states should be included in this group. Drugs that are known to be porphyrogenic in AIP, as well as those thought to be safe, are presented in Table 7.8 (Eales, 1979).

Acute attacks of AIP may affect many organ systems. Abdominal pain with a rigid abdomen is common, as are migrating, unusual central and peripheral neurologic findings which are often diagnosed as conversion disorders. At our hospital, we have seen patchy demyelination of the CNS, hypotension, and adult respiratory distress syndrome during a fulminant attack. Milder attacks almost certainly occur, which go unrecognized or are considered psychiatric events.

Psychiatric symptomatology is a prominent feature of the acute attacks in 50–75% of cases. Psychopathology may be common during the "'interictal" period as well. Ackner and colleagues (1962) have reviewed the somewhat sparse literature in this regard, as well as providing 13 cases they have studied. The psychiatric symptoms associated with the attacks are protean, but include agitation, which may be wild and violent or which may appear more anxious; nonparanoid psychotic features; and depressive features. In the few patients we have seen, we have had the impression of a global emotional instability which is experienced over a prolonged time course surrounding an attack. In Tishler *et al.*'s 1985 review of psychiatric symptoms among porphyric patients in a state hospital, a similar wide array of diagnoses were seen.

## Demographics

Autosomal-dominant inheritance characterizes AIP, but expression is more common among women. It is more common among people of Scandinavian origin, where prevalence rates for the gene may be 1/13,000. Clinical onset typically first occurs in early adult life.

## Clinical History

Have there been previous acute events characterized by agitation, anxiety, or psychosis? Abdominal pain? Neurologic events that were difficult to diagnose? Did any of these events coincide with menstrual cycle, infection, diet, or drug administration? Have there been diagnoses of conversion disorders? Is there a family history of neurologic or psychiatric disease?

---

*Clinical Rule 7.2:* Severe abdominal pain + madness of any sort = porphyria until proved otherwise

---

## Psychotropic Drug Interactions

**Benzodiazepines.** Probably safe, but experience is limited.

**Barbiturates.** All derivatives can precipitate attacks.

**Anticonvulsants.** Carbamazepine has a questionable status. Phenytoin and phenobarbital are definite precipitants.

**Antidepressants.** Probably safe (see Table 7.8).

## Mental Status Examination

There is anecdotal evidence that some AIP patients develop dementia, but good descriptions are not available.

## General Medical Examination

Between attacks there are no specific findings. During attacks a painful and rigid abdomen may be seen, along with occasional hypotension and acute respiratory distress syndrome (ARDS). Patients may become critically ill or die. Milder clinical attacks almost certainly occur and escape clinical detection.

## Neurological Examination

Neurologic deficits appear in some but not all patients. Once present, they may improve, but they often leave permanent residua. The pathophysiology seems to be acute demyelination, which may affect either proximal peripheral nerves or CNS. Brainstem findings have been common in our limited experience.

CNS. Check for nystagmus, disconjugate gaze, dysarthria, or other evidence of brainstem demyelination.

Sensory. The acute neuropathy is more motor than sensory, but we have observed sensory deficits as well. Check the four primary sensory modalities.

Motor. Check for flaccid weakness or atrophy.

Reflex. Both hyporeflexia and pathologic hyperreflexic can be seen, either acutely during an attack or as permanent residual deficits.

## Laboratory and Imaging (see Pathak and West, 1982)

Urine. Four precursor molecules may be assayed in a 24-hr urine:

| | Normal result |
|---|---|
| Delta-aminolevulinic acid | $< 4000\ \mu g$ |
| Porphobilinogen | $< 1500\ \mu g$ |
| Uroporphyrin | $< 40\ \mu g$ |
| Coproporphyrin | $< 280\ \mu g$ |

These assays may be *normal* between attacks. If the precursors are present, the urine may turn to a reddish or amber color upon standing in sunlight. The clinician cannot rely on this occurring, but it is diagnostic when it does.

Enzyme (in Blood). Fifty percent or greater reduction in porphobilinogen deaminase. This assay must usually be sent to a research laboratory, with control samples from normals.

## EPILEPSY-RELATED ANXIETY DISORDER

There are reports of anxietylike phenomena occurring in association with partial complex seizure disorders (Brodsky *et al.*, 1983). It may also be true that some patients with atypical panic attacks involving hostility, irritability, and derealization have abnormal EEGs (Edlund *et al.*, 1987). It has not been our experience, however, that many epileptics are misdiagnosed as panic–anxiety patients.

*Clinical Rule 7.3:* Where there are no seizures . . . there is no epilepsy.

## REFERENCES

Ackner, B., Cooper, J. E., Gray, C. H., and Kelly, M. Acute porphyria: A neuropsychiatric and biochemical study. *J. Psychosom. Res.*, 1962, **6,** 1–24.

Aronson, T. A., and Craig, T. J. Cocaine precipitation of panic disorders. *Am. J. Psychiatry*, 1986, **143,** 643–645.

Bowen, R. C., Orchard, R. C., Keegan, D. L., and D'Arcy, C. Mitral valve prolapse and psychiatric disorders. *Psychosomatics*, 1985, **26,** 926–932.

Bravo, E. L., Tarazi, R. C., Gifford, R. W., and Stewart, B. H. Circulatory and urinary catecholamines in pheochromocytoma: Diagnosis and pathophysiologic implications. *N. Engl. J. Med.* 1979, **301,** 682–686.

Breier, A., Charney, D. S., and Heninger, G. R. Major depression in patients with agoraphobia and panic disorder. *Arch. Gen. Psychiatry*, 1984, **41,** 1129–1135.

Brodsky, L., Zuniga, J. S., and Casenas, E. R. Refractory anxiety: A masked epileptiform disorder? *Psychiatr. M. Univ. Ottawa*, 1983, **8,** 42–45.

Carlson, R. J. Longitudinal observations of two cases of organic anxiety syndrome. *Psychosomatics*, 1986, **27,** 529–531.

Chopra, I. J., and Solomon, D. H. Pathogenesis of hyperthyroidism. *Annu. Rev. Med.*, 1983, **34,** 267–281.

Coyle, P. K., and Sterman, A. B. Focal neurologic symptoms in panic attacks. *Am. J. Psychiatry*, 1986, **143,** 648–649.

Crooks, J., Murray, I. P. C., and Wayne, E. J. Statistical methods applied to the clinical diagnosis of thyrotoxicosis. *Q. J. M.*, 1959, **28,** 211–234.

Denko, J. D., and Kaelbling, R. The psychiatric aspects of hypoparathyroidism. *Acta Psychiatr. Scand.*, 1962, **38** (Suppl. 164), 1–70.

*Diagnostic and Statistical Manual of Mental Disorders*, 3d ed., Rev. Washington, DC: American Psychiatric Association, 1987.

Dietch, J. T. Diagnosis of organic anxiety disorders. *Psychosomatics*, 1981, **22,** 661–669.

Eales, L. Porphyria and the dangerous life-threatening drugs. *S. Afr. Med. J.*, 1979, **56,** 914–917.

Edlund, M. J., Swann, A. C., and Clothier, J. Patients with panic attacks and abnormal EEG results. *Am. J. Psychiatry*, 1987, **144,** 508–509.

Goldfrank, L., and Starke, C. L. Metabolic acidosis in the alcoholic. *Hosp. Physician*, 1979, **14,** 34–37.

Gorman, J. M., Shear, M. K., Devereux, R. B., King, D. L., and Klein, D. F. Prevalence of mitral valve prolapse in panic disorder: Effect of echocardiographic criteria. *Psychosom. Med.*, 1986, **48,** 167–171.

Greden, J. F. Anxiety or caffeinism: A diagnostic dilemma. *Am. J. Psychiatry*, 1974, **131,** 1089–1092.

Greden, J. F., Fontaine, P., Lubetsky, M., and Chamberlin, K. Anxiety and depression associated with caffeinism among psychiatric inpatients. *Am. J. Psychiatry*, 1978, **135,** 963–966.

Hamburger, J. I. The various presentations of thyroiditis. Diagnostic considerations. *Ann. Intern. Med.*, 1986, **104,** 219–224.

Heinik, J. Hyperthyroidism and the organic anxiety syndrome. *Am. J. Psychiatry*, 1986, **143,** 1497–1498 (letter).

Hoehn-Saric, R. Neurotransmitters in anxiety. *Arch. Gen. Psychiatry*, 1982, **39,** 735–742.

Hoffman, W. H., Chodoroff, G., and Piggott, L. R. Haloperidol and thyroid storm. *Am. J. Psychiatry*, 1978, **135,** 484–486.

Hurley, J. R. Thyroid disease in the elderly. *Med. Clin. North Am.*, 1983, **67,** 497–516.

Jefferson, J. W., and Marshall, J. R. *Neuropsychiatric Features of Medical Disorders*. New York: Plenum Press, 1981, p. 4.

Kaplan, M. M., and Utiger, R. D. Diagnosis of hyperthyroidism. *Clin. Endocrinol. Metab.*, 1978, **7,** 97–113.

Kathol, R. G., Turner, R., and Delahunt, J. Depression and anxiety associated with hyperthyroidism: Response to antithyroid therapy. *Psychosomatics*, 1986, **27,** 501–505.

Leckman, J. F., Merikangas, K. R., Pauls, D. L., Prusoff, B. A., and Weismann, M. M. Anxiety disorders and depression: Contradictions between family study data and DSM III conventions. *Am. J. Psychiatry*, 1983, **140,** 880–882.

Levine, R. Hypoglycemia. *JAMA*, 1974, **230,** 462–463.

Liberthson, R., Sheehan, D. V., King, M. E., and Weyman, A. E. The prevalance of mitral valve prolapse in patients with panic disorders. *Am. J. Psychiatry*, 1986, **143,** 511–515.

Maturzas, W., Al-Sadir, J., Uhlenhuth, E. H., and Glass, R. M. Mitral valve prolapse and thyroid abnormalities in patients with panic attacks. *Am. J. Psychiatry*, 1987, **144,** 493–496.

May, P. R. A., and Ebaugh, F. G. Pathological intoxication, alcoholic hallucinosis, and other reactions to alcohol: A clinical study. *Q. J. Stud. Alcohol*, 1953, **14,** 200–227.

Mazza, D. L., Martin, D., Spacavento, L., Jacobsen, J., and Gibbs, H. Prevalence of anxiety disorders in patients with mitral valve prolapse. *Am. J. Psychiatry*, 1986, **143,** 349–352.

Medical Letter. Drugs that cause psychiatric symptoms. *Med. Lett. Drugs Ther.*, 1986, **28,** 81–86.

*Mental Disorders: Glossary and Guide to Their Classification in Accordance with the Ninth Revision of the International Classification of Diseases*. Geneva: World Health Organization, 1978.

Miles, W. R. The comparative concentration of alcohol in human blood and urine at intervals after ingestion. *J. Pharmacol. Exp. Ther.*, 1922, **20,** 265.

New England Journal of Medicine. Table of normal reference laboratory values. *N. Engl. J. Med.*, 1986, **314,** 39–49.

Nishimura, R. A., McGoon, M. D., Shub, C., Miller, F. A., Ilstrup, D. M., and Tajik, A. J.

Echocardiographically documented mitral-valve prolapse: Long-term follow-up of 237 patients. *N. Engl. J. Med.*, 1985, **313,** 1305–1309.
Pathak, M. A., and West, J. D. Porphyrias: Office procedures and laboratory tests for diagnosis of porphyrin abnormalities. *Acta Derma. Venereol.* (Stockh.), 1982, **100** (Suppl.), 91–105.
Rosenman, R. H. The impact of anxiety on the cardiovascular system. *Psychosomatics*, 1985, **26** (Suppl. 11), 6–15.
Savage, D. D., Garrison, R. J., Devereux, R. B., Castelli, W. P., Anderson, S. J., Levy, D., McNamara, P. M., Stokes, K., Kannel, W. B., and Feinleib, M. Mitral valve prolapse in the general population. I. Epidemiologic features: The Framingham Study. *Am. Heart J.*, 1983, **106,** 571–576.
Schuckit, M. A. Anxiety related to medical disease. *J. Clin. Psychiatry*, 1983, **44,** 31–36.
Shader, R. I. Panic disorders: Epidemiologic and family studies. *Psychosomatics*, 1984, **25** (Suppl. 10), 10–15.
Shader, R. I., Goodman, M., and Gever, J. Panic disorders: Current perspectives. *J. Clin. Psychopharmacol.*, 1982, **2** (Suppl. 6), 25–105.
Starkman, M. N., Zelnik, T. C., Nesse, R. M., and Cameron, O. G. Anxiety in patients with pheochromocytomas. *Arch. Intern. Med.*, 1985, **145,** 248–252.
Stein, M. B. Panic disorder and medical illness. *Psychosomatics*, 1986, **27,** 833–838.
Szmuilowicz, J., and Flannery, J. G. Mitral valve prolapse syndrome and psychological disturbance. *Psychosomatics*, 1980, **21,** 419–421.
Tishler, P. V., Woodward, B., O'Connor, J., Holbrook, D. A., Seidman, L. J., Hallett, M., and Knighton, D. J. High prevalence of intermittent acute porphyria in a psychiatric patient population. *Am. J. Psychiatry*, 1985, **142,** 1430–1436.
Tschudy, D. P., Valsamis, M., and Magnussen, C. R. Acute intermittent porphyria: Clinical and selected research aspects. *Ann. Intern. Med.*, 1975, **183,** 851–864.
Weiner, M. F. Haloperidol, hyperthyroidism, and sudden death. *Am. J. Psychiatry*, 1979, **136,** 717–718.
Weissman, M. M., Myers, J. K., and Harding, P. S. Psychiatric disorders in a U.S. urban community, 1975–1976. *Am. J. Psychiatry*, 1978, **135,** 459–462.
Williams, L. C., Turney, J. H., and Parsons, V. Beta blocker withdrawal syndrome. *Lancet*, 1979, **1,** 94–95 (letter).
Wilson, W. H., and Jefferson, J. W. Thyroid disease, behavior, and psychopharmacology. *Psychosomatics*, 1985, **26,** 481–492.
Witschy, J. K., and Redmond, F. C. Extrapyramidal reaction to fluphenazine potentiated by thyrotoxicosis. *Am. J. Psychiatry*, 1981, **138,** 246–247.
Wynne, J. Mitral valve prolapse. *N. Engl. J. Med.*, 1986, **314,** 577–578 (letter).

# 8

# Paranoid Psychosis

## DSM-III-R-Diagnoses

*Paranoid Schizophrenia.* A type of schizophrenia in which there are:

1. Preoccupation with one or more systematized delusions or with frequent auditory hallucinations related to a single theme.
2. None of the following: incoherence, marked loosening of association, flat or grossly inappropriate affect, catatonic behavior, grossly disorganized behavior.

*Delusional Paranoid Disorders.* The presence of a persistent, nonbizarre delusion that is not due to any other mental disorder. The delusion(s) typically involves situations that occur in real life, such as being followed, infected, loved at a distance, having a disease, or being deceived by one's spouse or lover.

*Paranoid Personality Disorder.* A pervasive and unwarranted tendency, beginning by early adulthood and present in a variety of contexts, to interpret the actions of people as deliberately demeaning or threatening.

## ICD-9 Diagnoses

*Paranoid Schizophrenia.* The form of schizophrenia in which relatively stable delusions, which may be accompanied by hallucinations, dominate the clinical picture. The delusions are frequently of persecution but may take other forms (for example of jealousy, exalted birth, Messianic mission, or bodily change). Hallucinations and erratic behavior may occur; in some cases conduct is seriously disturbed from the outset, thought disorder may be gross, and affective flattening with fragmentary delusions and hallucinations may develop.

*Paranoid State, Simple.* A psychosis, acute or chronic, not classifiable as schizophrenia or affective psychosis, in which delusions, especially of being influenced, persecuted or treated in some special way, are the main symptoms. The delusions are of a fairly fixed, elaborate and systematized kind.

*Paranoia.* A rare chronic psychosis in which logically constructed systematized delusions have developed gradually without concomitant hallucinations or the schizophrenic type of disordered thinking. The delusions are mostly of grandeur (the paranoiac prophet or inventor), persecution, or somatic abnormality.

*Paraphrenia.* Paranoid psychosis in which there are conspicuous hallucinations, often in several modalities. Affective symptoms and disordered thinking, if present, do not dominate the clinical picture and the personality is well preserved.

In each of our psychiatric syndrome-related chapters thus far, we have discussed drug-induced syndromes first and epilepsy last. We are forced to reverse this approach for the paranoid disorders. The issue of the link between paranoia and epilepsy overshadows clinical research interest in other medically based paranoid states. This may be understandable from a research point of view, but clinically it can be a very limited perspective from which to view the paranoias. In approaching the diagnostic evaluation of any paranoid condition, we are quite sympathetic with the general principles enunciated by Anderson (1979):

1. Retain a high index of suspicion for "organic" brain disease.
2. Beware of jumping to the conclusion that acute psychosis is schizophrenia or manic-depressive disorder because the patient has recently experienced a psychologic or social "precipitating event."
3. Beware of assuming that acute psychosis is schizophrenia or manic-depressive disorders because of specific mental content or symptoms.
4. The more rapid the onset of acute psychosis, the more likely it is to be "organic."
5. Schizophrenia and mania typically begin before age 40.
6. Acute psychosis in patients who have serious medical illness usually results from complications of the illness itself or its treatment.

A wide array of medical and neurologic diseases have been reported to occur in association with paranoid psychotic features (for a review, see Davison and Bagley, 1969). The clinical research limitations that have beset us in other chapters recur here: many of the reports are anecdotal; control groups are few; and clinical details of the psychotic states themselves are sparse. The paranoid disorders present yet an additional difficulty for the clinician. Those paranoid conditions that have been considered psychogenic occur across a wide range of life-span, from childhood schizophrenia to the paraphrenias. Many of the medical–neurologic disorders that may be confounded with such conditions also

**Table 8.1**
Medical–Neurologic Diseases Associated with Acute Paranoid States

| | |
|---|---|
| Partial complex epilepsy | Drugs and toxins |
| Trauma | Cocaine |
| Tumor | Marijuana |
| Stroke | Bronchodilators |
| Degenerative diseases | Alcohol |
| Alzheimer's disease | Amphetamines |
| Parkinson's disease | Anticholinergics |
| Narcolepsy | L-dopa |
| Paraphrenia | Isoniazid |
| Huntington's disease | Benzodiazepines |
| | Ephedrine |
| | Bromocriptine |
| | Infection |
| | Metabolic (few) |

span human development widely. Demographic clues are less useful in this clinical area. One has to have a sense of those relatively few disorders that are truly *likely* to be interspersed within a paranoid population and how to recognize them. The categories of such disorders we propose to discuss in this chapter are listed in Table 8.1.

What is the frequency of association between paranoid mental states and these various syndromes? How closely do the paranoid states associated with these conditions mimic the major psychiatric paranoias? We just do not know with certainty. In their 1969 review, Davison and Bagley attempted to construct a "retrospective epidemiologic" study, using frequencies of reported CNS disorders among groups of psychotic patients and comparing them with expected frequencies among the population at large (see Table 8.2). It is noteworthy from this compilation that frequencies of epilepsy among psychotic patients did *not* exceed expectations, despite the purported connection between partial complex epilepsy and paranoia (a connection we do not dispute).

## TEMPORAL LOBE EPILEPSY

A 26-year-old man was referred to psychiatric clinic for evaluation and treatment of a paranoid disorder. He had experienced ideas of reference since late adolescence, along with episodic persecutory auditory hallucinations. His mother stated that he occasionally appeared inexplicably "groggy" or "like a drunk," and his face twitched. A discharging focus was present on EEG across the medial side of the left temporal lobe.

**Table 8.2**
Relative Risk for Psychosis among Various Medical–Neurologic Diseases[a,b]

| CNS disorder | Prevalence in general population (per 100,000) | Distribution of psychotic cases in 1958–1967 literature | |
|---|---|---|---|
| | | Expected number | Actual number[c] |
| Trauma | — | — | 532 |
| Epilepsy | 548 | 211 | 276 |
| Huntington's chorea | 4 | 2 | 86* |
| Cerebrovascular disease | 450 | 173 | 42* |
| Parkinsonism | 114 | 44 | 20* |
| Narcolepsy | — | — | 19* |
| Choreoathetosis | — | — | 19 |
| Cerebral glioma | 8.3 | 3 | 19* |
| Benign cerebral tumor | 30 | 12 | 17 |
| Pituitary adenoma | 5.4 | 2 | 17* |
| Post meningitis/encephalitis | — | — | 16 |
| Multiple sclerosis | 80 | 30 | 11* |
| Congenital disorders | — | — | 8 |
| General paresis | 24 | 9 | 5 |
| Hepatic encephalopathy | — | — | 5 |
| Wilson's disease | — | — | 4 |
| Cerebellar degeneration | 7 | 3 | 3 |
| Other cerebral degeneration | — | — | 3 |
| Cerebral lipoidosis | — | — | 3 |
| Hypoglycemia | — | — | 3 |
| Motor neuron disease | 11 | 4 | 2 |
| Cerebral reticulosis | — | — | 2 |
| Torsion spasm | — | — | 2 |
| Leber's optic atrophy | — | — | 1 |
| Phenylketonuria | — | — | 1 |
| Schilder's disease | — | — | 1 |
| Friedreich's ataxia | — | — | 1 |
| Myotonia congenita | — | — | 1 |

[a]Comparison of the relative proportion of CNS disorders with psychosis in the 1958–1967 literature and their prevalence in the general population.
[b]Reprinted from Davison and Bagley (1969), with permission.
[c]Indicates probable significant difference.

It is difficult to escape the conclusion that an association of some kind exists between temporal lobe epilepsy and paranoid psychotic states. Although a few authors remain skeptical (e.g., Stevens, 1966; Stevens and Herman, 1981), the weight of evidence for such an association as detailed in several recent reviews seems incontrovertible (see Slater, 1969; Blumer, 1975; Trimble, 1984; 1985; Pincus and Tucker, 1985; McKenna *et al.*, 1985). In our view, the areas of genuine controversy and active research have shifted from the association itself to second-order issues, including the quality and natural history of the epileptiform psychoses, mechanisms underlying the association, treatment issues, and others.

In considering these epileptiform psychoses, it is important to have a conceptual framework by which to organize them. First, it is important to be reminded of the range of the clinical epilepsies. Although partial seizures with complex symptomatology have been the focus of most research concerning psychosis and paranoia, there are several other types of seizures. The present classification proposed by the International League against Epilepsy is presented in Table 8.3.

Of course, alterations of mental status functions may occur during and after seizure types other than partial complex seizures. In particular, absence-like seizures and status epilepticus may present with a disorganized, psychotic picture (we discuss this in Chapter 9). It is the partial complex of seizures, however, that have been linked on a clinical basis with paranoid states. Most

**Table 8.3**
International Classification of Epileptic Seizures

I. Partial seizures (seizures beginning locally)
   A. Partial seizures with elementary symptomatology (generally without impairment of consciousness)
      1. With motor symptoms (includes jacksonian seizures)
      2. With special sensory symptoms
      3. With autonomic symptoms
      4. Compound forms
   B. Partial seizures with complex symptomatology (generally with impairment of consciousness)
      1. With impairment of consciousness only
      2. With cognitive symptomatology
      3. With affective symptomatology
      4. With "psychosensory" symptomatology
      5. With "psychomotor" symptomatology (automatisms)
      6. Compound forms
   C. Partial seizures secondarily generalized
II. Generalized seizures (bilaterally symmetric and without local onset)
   1. Absences *(petit mal)*
   2. Bilateral massive epileptic myoclonus
   3. Infantile spasms
   4. Clonic seizures
   5. Tonic seizures
   6. Tonic–clonic seizures *(grand mal)*
   7. Atonic seizures
   8. Akinetic seizures
III. Unilateral seizures
IV. Unclassified epileptic seizures

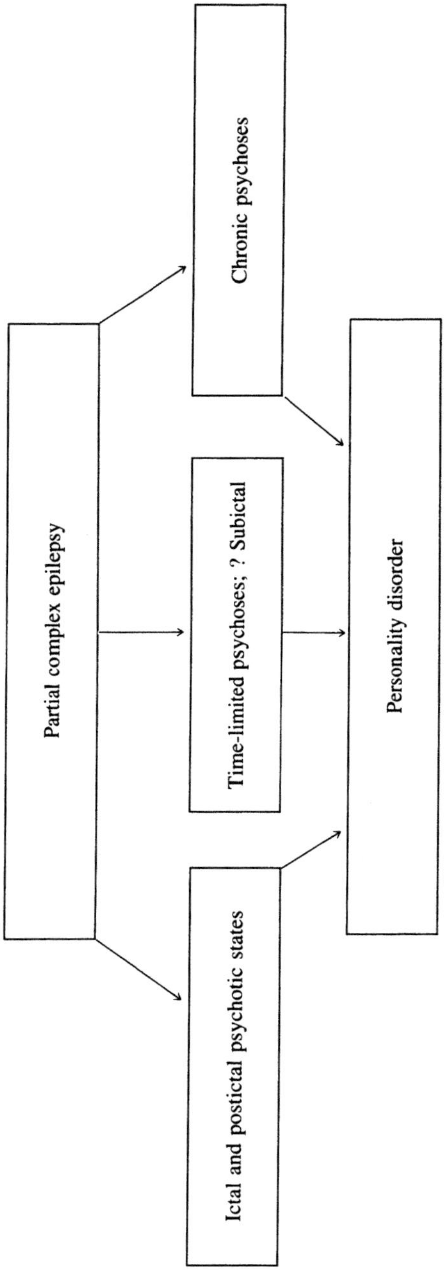


**Figure 8.1.** Psychoses associated with temporal lobe epilepsy.

of these seizures have a temporal lobe focus or foci, although some have mesial frontal lobe foci. This is the most common of the adult epilepsies. We will direct the remainder of our discussion to this problem.

Within the clinical area of patients who have both partial complex epilepsy and a psychosis, one needs a conceptual scheme by which to organize the data. We propose the outline depicted in Fig. 8.1.

We are suggesting that the epileptiform psychoses be organized according to their relationship with the seizures themselves. Such a classification scheme provides a useful solution to a psychiatric issue of increasing controversy—the nonepileptiform psychotic patient who has an abnormal EEG. Despite the value of the EEG during the diagnostic evaluation of "spells," it remains only confirmatory with regard to the diagnosis of epilepsy. This diagnosis remains essentially a clinical judgment. Patients may be considered epileptic, despite a normal EEG, when the clinician judges that they have seizures. If a patient has no seizures, one should not consider him epileptic. In a large series of psychiatric inpatients, one can expect 2.6% to have epileptiform EEGs without a clinical history of seizures (Bridgers, 1987). These people do not have epilepsy. Until more extensive clinical research appears, we recommend that they *not* be classified according to our schema and *not* diagnosed "TLE psychosis."

---

*Clinical Rule 8.1:* Where there are no seizures, there is no epilepsy.

---

## Ictal and Postictal Paranoid Psychoses

Those clinical phenomena that contribute to the syndrome we recognize as a paranoid psychotic state—grandiose feelings, ideas of reference, complex auditory hallucinations—do *not* typically arise directly from ictal discharges or from immediate postictal states. This is not to say that alterations of visual, sensory, auditory, and emotional experience may not occur as part of a complex seizure, for they commonly do. But the quality and context of these clinical events are such that they can usually be recognized as epileptic.

More than half of the patients with partial complex epilepsy surveyed by Williams (1956) stated that alterations of emotional state could occur as part of their seizures. The most common of these emotional experiences included a variety of dysphoric and unpleasant emotions; sudden fears, dreads, frights, and sadnesses. Typically, these sudden alterations of mood occurred early in the evolution of a partial complex seizure, probably during the focal onset portion of the seizure, and they were brief, lasting seconds. Currie and associates (1971) interviewed 666 patients with partial complex epilepsy and found that 19% reported emotional alterations during their seizures. As in the report of Williams, these authors described a vast preponderance of unpleasant emotions among these patients. Hermann *et al.* (1982) have suggested that epileptic patients who experience ictal fear early in their complex seizures may constitute a subgroup of seizure patients at greater risk for development of paranoid psychoses and other psychopathology.

A variety of hallucinatory and illusionary experiences may occur as ictal phenomena, most commonly in the context of a more elaborate partial complex seizure. One need only consider that the temporal lobe contains relay and processing mechanisms for all five of the primary sensory modalities in order to imagine the variety of ictal sensory experiences that may occur. In the large series of patients cited by Currie *et al.* (1971), ictal alterations of sensory modalities occurred with the following frequencies: visual, 18%; auditory, 16%; olfactory, 12%; gustatory, 3%; sensory, 2%. The majority of these hallucinations are crude or ineffable alterations of sensory experience, as opposed to formed, "psychoticlike" hallucinations (Simpson, 1969). Unpleasant odors, flashing lights, distortions of sound, or "noises like rushing water"—these sorts of experience are not usually confused with psychotic symptomatology. When more integrated auditory hallucinations do occur as ictal events, they tend to be repetitive and stereotypical. In Williams's report (1956), for example, one man is described who experienced the sound of the announcer for the 9 o'clock news as the herald for many of his seizures.

An additional, important quality that characterizes most behavioral disturbances associated with ictal discharge is that they are accompanied by an alteration of consciousness (Goldensohn and Gold, 1960). These patients appear "dreamy," "spacy," "confused." Movements that occur tend to be repetitive and stereotypical. This confused and disorganized quality also characterizes the immediate postictal period, which may last from minutes to hours or even days. Specific psychotic symptoms may not be elicited during this period because of the patient's obtundation and disorganization. They may "appear" quite assaultive and uncontrollable, however, particularly if efforts are made to restrain them (Special Report, 1981).

## Time-Limited Epileptic Psychoses

There are reports of brief paranoid–hallucinatory states occurring among patients with partial complex epilepsy in which no alteration or disorganization of consciousness is seen (Landolt, 1953; Dongier, 1959/1960). Concurrent EEG tracings were available for many of the brief psychotic episodes described in these reports, which showed no evidence of epileptiform discharge. Corroboration of these older studies using current clinical and electrophysiologic techniques would be of great interest because of the possibility that these brief psychoses in clear consciousness represent confined limbic-system discharges. We have clinically observed such brief psychotic episodes occurring after a flurry of partial complex seizures that have been quickly brought under medical control. Such psychoses may also represent a variant of the phenomenon that has been labeled "forced normalization," or the sudden appearance of psychosis with normal EEG after cessation of a series of seizures (Pakalnis *et al.*, 1987). Further clinical research is needed in this area.

## Chronic Epileptic Psychoses

Despite isolated dissenting opinions, there is a preponderant clinical research literature indicating an association between partial complex (probably temporal lobe) epilepsy and chronic schizophreniform psychoses (see reviews cited earlier). A predominance of paranoid/hallucinatory clinical presentations is described in these reports, although less frequent descriptions of atypical catatonic psychoses also appear. In general, these psychotic states tend to develop after several years of seizure occurrence, as if some neurophysiologic change related to chronic seizure discharge were a prerequisite for the psychosis. Patients with very good seizure control are less likely to develop the syndrome. A variety of somewhat unusual behaviors may accompany the psychosis, including hypergraphia, hyperreligiosity, a "viscous" emotional quality, and others. There may be a correlation between the paranoid version of this chronic epileptic psychosis and a left hemisphere seizure focus (Sherwin *et al.*, 1982). There may be a correlation between presence of psychosis and cognitive impairments. An important question for clinicians concerns how nearly these epilepsy-associated paranoid psychoses might mimic "true" paranoid schizophrenia. Some carefully done studies using standardized interviews and appropriate comparison groups have found identical clinical profiles between the epileptic psychoses and the schizophrenic psychoses (Perez and Trimble, 1980; Toone *et al.*, 1982). Other observers have stressed some distinctive qualities of the epileptic paranoid states, with greater preservation of affect, interpersonal relatedness, and functional status than in the schizophrenic paranoias (Slater *et al.*, 1963; Stoudemire *et al.*, 1983).

Our clinical experience has tended to support both sides of this issue. We have seen some epileptic patients who were indistinguishable from schizophrenics but for their seizures. We have also seen several individuals whose epileptic psychoses seemed more "encapsulated," with greater preservation of affective responsiveness and psychosocial relatedness than might have been expected in a schizophreniform disorder.

It is important to stress that all of the patients we have been referring to, as well as those described in the reports cited, were patients who had definite *seizures*. Some partial complex seizures are more obvious clinically than others, but the evidence for epilepsy in an individual usually becomes manifest during the usual course of history, examination, and observation. Abnormal

EEGs alone do not diagnose epilepsy. The notion of paranoid psychosis associated with "subclinical epilepsy" is an unproven one. At the risk of being proved wrong by future research, we would observe that such a concept has not been a clinically useful one in our experience. The primary difficulty in postulating "subclinical epilepsy" in patients with chronic psychoses is the relatively high rate of abnormal EEGs seen among schizophrenics. Without clinical seizures, it becomes difficult to identify the epileptics.

## Checkpoints—Epilepsy and Paranoia

### Demographics

Partial seizures with complex symptomatology are the most common of the adult epilepsies, with a lifetime risk as high as 0.3% (Gastaut *et al.*, 1975). More than 50% of first seizures occur after age 25, and onset in older patients with stroke or tumor is common. There is no sexual predilection. The most common neuropathologies include mesial temporal sclerosis (presumably related to congenital or early-life injury), stroke, tumor, trauma, and hamartoma. Patients who have had any of the above diseases are at greater risk for developing epilepsy and, presumably, the epileptic psychoses.

### Clinical History

It is not surprising that there are patients with character pathology who wish to be considered epileptic; it is surprising that there are patients with true partial complex epilepsy who do not know they have it. Paranoid epileptic patients are usually obviously epileptic with more subtle paranoia; occasionally some are seen who are obviously paranoid and more subtly epileptic. As is often the case in clinical medicine, the history is of greater importance than the examination.

When asking after the clinical history of epilepsy, it is important to remember major risk-conferring events that may occur in early life. Did the patient experience birth trauma or birth injury? Were there unusually high fevers during childhood or febrile seizures? Has there been significant head injury? Has there been meningitis or encephalitis? Is there a family history for epilepsy (not that partial complex is a heritable form of epilepsy, but this may indicate the patient's familiarity with seizures).

When asking about seizures themselves, it is important to use a variety of terms as value-neutral as possible. Many people would be scandalized to admit to "fits" or "convulsions," but are quite willing to describe "spells" they have experienced. Sometimes people will acknowledge "faints" or "falls" but not "seizures." Ask the patient to describe any spells carefully. Syncope is not

| | |
|---|---|
| Haloperidol | Highest |
| Thioridazine | ↑ |
| Chlorpromazine | |
| Fluphenazine | |
| Thioridazine | |
| Pimozide | |
| Molindone | Lowest |

**Figure 8.2.** Relative ranking of antipsychotic drugs for epileptogenic potential.

epilepsy; nor is depersonalization, hyperventilation, light-headedness, vertigo, or headache. For patients who acknowledge generalized tonic or clonic seizures, ask carefully concerning any aura that may precede them, thereby classifying them as partial complex. Strange gastrointestinal sensations and odors are particularly common at the onset of seizures with temporal lobe foci.

Temporal lobe seizures are particularly likely to occur or exacerbate at onset of sleep or during sleep. Ask the patients if they wet the bed at night, bite their tongues, stir the bedclothes in a remarkable way, or bounce around so as to disturb sleeping partners.

## Psychotropic–Anticonvulsant Drug Interactions

Group I. Antipsychotic–antiepileptic drug interactions occur and are probably of sufficient magnitude to be of clinical significance in some cases. More research is needed in this area. Carbamazepine, for example, has been the subject of very few reports with regard to such interactions. Phenobarbital, phenytoin, and most antipsychotic drugs probably mutually compete for and induce the hepatic cytochrome P-450 enzyme system (Linnoila *et al.*, 1980; Woodbury *et al.*, 1982; Gay and Madsen, 1983). [The reduction in serum haloperidol levels that can be induced by carbamazepine has been shown to be clinically significant in some patients (Arana *et al.*, 1986).] In general, one should expect a diminution of serum level for any given drug dosage when these anticonvulsants are used in combination with antipsychotics. Plasma levels and clinical efficacy of antipsychotic drugs may be reduced in turn.

Group II. An additional, less "direct" interaction between antipsychotic and antiepileptic drugs is mediated by the antipsychotic drugs' ability to lower seizure threshold on their own. All of the major tranquilizers are probably epileptogenic to some extent (Mendez *et al.*, 1984). The risk is dosage-related. It may be that as many as 10% of nonepileptic patients taking more than 100 mg chlorpromazine per day (or its equivalent) will experience a single seizure (Logothetis, 1967). In studies using *in vitro* models of epilepsy, a rank order of epileptogenic potential has been established for several common antipsychotic drugs (Fig. 8.2) (Oliver *et al.*, 1982).

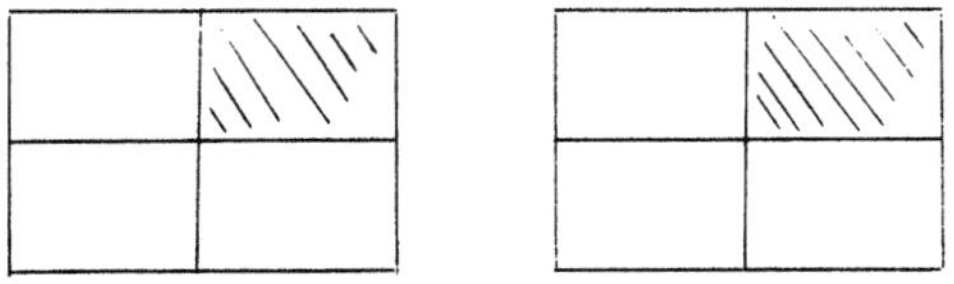

**Figure 8.3.** Visual-field defect from lesion of left temporal lobe.

Clinical experience, however, dictates that the epileptogenic potential of these drugs can almost always be compensated by adjustments in the anticonvulsant regimens.

---

*Clinical Rule 8.2:* There is no epileptic patient who cannot take some dose of one antipsychotic drug.

---

## Mental Status Examination

**Arousal.** Should be unimpaired, unless there has been recent seizure activity. Observe for brief lapses of attention and concentration during the interview, which may be seizure-related.

**Language.** The temporal lobes are the repository for most receptive language functions. Fully developed aphasia syndromes may be seen in some persons with temporal lobe lesions. An examination for *anomia* may be a sensitive if nonlocalizing clue to temporal lobe dysfunction.

**Interpersonal Relatedness.** There probably is a "retained relatedness" among some epileptic paranoid patients, which distinguishes them from some schizophrenics. It is unwise to place much diagnostic weight on this feature.

## General Medical Examination

No abnormalities specific to temporal lobe epilepsy.

## Neurological Examination

In general, the temporal lobes are "silent" on the neurologic examination when the mental status is omitted. One useful bit of neuroanatomy to keep in mind is that the inferior portion of the optic radiations (Meyer's loop) arcs through the central portion of the temporal lobes. Any lesion large enough to injure this loop can produce a contralateral homonymous, superior quadrantanopsia (see Fig. 8.3). This finding must be looked for more carefully than by brief finger confrontation. A 3-mm red-target may be necessary, with separate testing of each eye.

## Laboratory Tests

EEG. EEG is at once the most helpful and the most troublesome of tests related to paranoid psychosis. It represents the archetypal sensitive but nonspecific laboratory test. Two clinical rules are important:

---

*Clinical Rule 8.3:* Schizophrenic patients have abnormal EEGs.

*Clinical Rule 8.4*: Abnormal EEG $\neq$ epilepsy.

---

A wide variety of EEG abnormalities, including hemispheric asymmetries, abnormal fast frequencies, irregular rhythms, and even sharp forms, have been reported in schizophrenics (Hughes and Wilson, 1983). The explanation for these abnormalities is not known, but they do not make these patients into epileptics. Similarly, interictal epileptogenic discharges on EEG do not make the diagnosis of epilepsy, since some normal persons have such abnormalities (Delgado-Escueta, 1979). Indeed, some epileptic patients demonstrate normal EEGs, especially when reliance is made on a single tracing. Epilepsy is a clinical diagnosis; the EEG is a laboratory test.

When one performs an EEG in the diagnostic evaluation of partial complex epilepsy, the abnormality one is looking for may look like the tracing shown in Fig. 8.4.

There is currently debate and disagreement as to whether an EEG with nasopharyngeal (NP) leads is more sensitive in picking up medial temporal lobe foci than is a regular EEG. One can read reports in favor of NP leads (Rovit *et al.*, 1961; Pampiglione and Kerridge, 1956) and against them (Neufeld *et al.*, 1986; Ramani *et al.*, 1985). Even if most temporal lobe epileptics will show some abnormalities on routine scalp leads, we suspect that medial temporal discharges are at least better seen on the sphenoidal leads. We currently obtain a nasopharyngeal EEG with natural or drug-induced sleep for this work-up.

CT/MR Scan. Every patient with a confirmed diagnosis of partial complex epilepsy deserves a CT or MR scan at least once during his or her clinical course, in our opinion. Paranoia per se does not merit a scan, nor does schizophrenia. The lesion one is seeking is the medial temporal area, and MR is the preferred test.

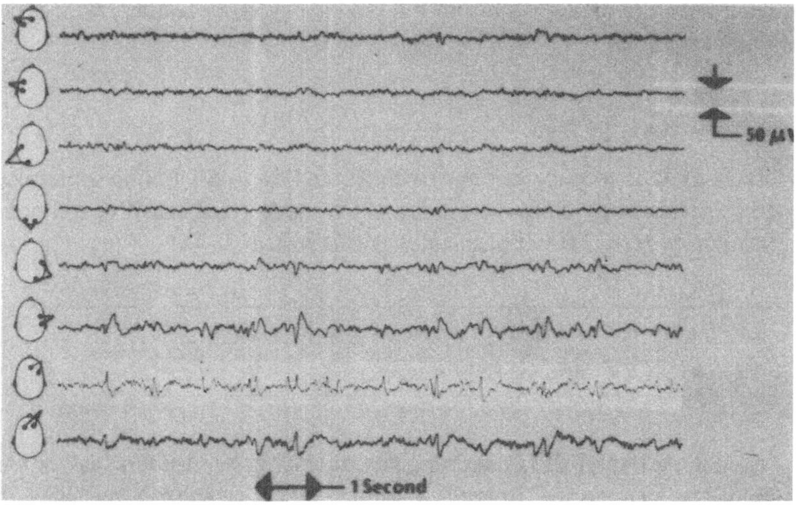


**Figure 8.4.** Interictal focal discharge in partial complex epilepsy.

## DRUGS AND TOXINS

A 31-year-old man was brought from jail to the psychiatry emergency room. He had a history of previous arrests for breaking and entering, but when he was picked up on this occasion the police noticed that he was acting "eccentric." On mental status examination he muttered continuously about "being the prophet," and he declaimed his fears that the "Philistines were coming to destroy the prophet." He complained of auditory hallucinations and demonstrated some stereotypical posturing of arms and neck which he stated to be religious rituals.

The list of drugs and toxins in Table 8.1 that have been associated with paranoid psychotic states is, again, somewhat misleading. Not all of these compounds are equally "suspicious." The closer the clinical picture is to an acute or chronic paranoid schizophreniform condition, the more likely it is that dopamine agonists (amphetamine, L-dopa, Sinemet, amantadine) are involved. Cocaine is another commonly used drug that is capable of manipulating the catecholamine system. We would suppose that almost any drug or toxin, if given in great enough dosage to a vulnerable person, would be capable of producing a delirious mental state that might have paranoid features. However, in such situations the "toxic encephalopathy" dimensions of the clinical picture or history are usually evident. This may not be true in the case of catecholaminergic agonists.

The amphetamines are panadrenergic agents ($\alpha$ and $\beta$ agonists; noradrenergic as well as dopaminergic) that are effective after oral dosing. They typically produce signs of heightened arousal and activation along with signs of diffuse sympathetic activation including elevated heart rate and systolic blood pressure, and diaphoresis and tremor. Single doses as low as 55 mg have been reported to cause acute, time-limited paranoid conditions (Connell, 1958). Paranoid schizophreniform states also emerge during the course of more prolonged abuse of drugs in this family, and this is the more common situation (Bell, 1965). The clinical picture typically includes ideas of reference, paranoid delusions, and auditory and visual hallucinations in a clear sensorium with intact orientation. Hyperactive deep tendon reflexes and dilated pupils are not, in our experience, features that help to distinguish the condition from schizophrenia, since they are sometimes common to both. We concur with Shader's conclusion that one cannot distinguish amphetamine psychosis from schizophrenia on clinical grounds (Shader, 1972). It is clear that other dopamine agonists including bromocriptine may induce similar mental states (Taneli *et al.*, 1986).

Cocaine, especially in its highly smokable form called "crack," is capable of inducing acute psychoses often characterized by aggression and paranoia (Medical Letter, 1986). Cocaine, too, is a CNS catecholamine agonist which produces increased heart rate and systolic blood pressure. It may also include hyperpyrexia, seizures, and ventricular arrhythmias. The cocaine-induced psychosis, similar to other catechol-related psychoses, may onset acutely after a single drug usage, or it may appear more insidiously among chronic heavy users.

Hallucinations and paranoid states occur in the course of long-term alcohol abuse, usually during withdrawal or partial withdrawal phases. Victor and Hope (1958) reported that 6% of 266 consecutive hospitalized alcoholics had auditory hallucinations in a clear sensorium. When they studied 76 of such patients with greater care, they found that only eight of them demonstrated a paranoid delusional system in addition to the hallucinosis. In most of these cases, the severity and chronicity of the alcoholism were such that metabolic, hepatic, and nutritional medical problems were obvious. Others have reported cases of alcohol-associated paranoia that were occasionally difficult to separate from paranoid schizophrenia (Sabot *et al.*, 1968; Hackett, 1978). More recently, similar phenomena have been reported in association with chronic, heavy benzodiazepine use, and with benzodiazepine withdrawal (Fraser and Ingram, 1985; Roberts and Vass, 1986). We suggest that CNS catecholamine excess associated with chronic or sudden withdrawal of such CNS depressants is the pathophysiologic mechanisms of these psychoses.

Anticholinergic drugs are another group of commonly used medications which have been reported in association with toxic paranoid states (see Stephens, 1967, for a review). In our experience there are two situations in which this is likely to occur. When anticholinergics are given to elderly patients or patients with metabolically compromised cerebral function, a toxic delirium with paranoid features may develop. The second situation may be that of psychotic young males who developed dystonias for which anticholinergics are added to their medical regimens. If the psychosis deepens secondary to the anticholinergic drugs, a vicious cycle may ensue, with parallel escalation of anticholinergic drugs and psychosis. In both of these situations, however, the physical stigmata of anticholinergic encephalopathy, including dry membranes, tachycardia, facial flushing, and ileus have been obvious upon examination.

One last group of compounds that may have some specificity with regard to their association with paranoid states is the bronchodilators, including theophylline, aminophylline, ephedrine, and others (Kane and Florenzano, 1971; Whitehouse and Duncan, 1987). Such patients typically have a history of bronchospasm, and on examination they demonstrate many of the hyperadrenergic signs seen in patients taking catecholamine agonists. We suspect that the bronchodilators are working at the level of the "second messenger" by elevating levels of cyclic AMP.

There are few other drugs or toxins that are likely to be encountered among paranoid patients. In the older literature, bromides were described as producing schizophreniform conditions (Levin, 1948). Marijuana (Talbott and Teague, 1969), isoniazid, carbon monoxide, and other compounds have been the subject of anecdotal research reports in this area. Most of these reports concerned clinical features that were admixed with encephalopathy.

## Checkpoints—Drugs and Toxins in Paranoid States

### Demographics

Amphetamine abuse may be more common among young males, and young people with patterns of drug abuse. Prevalence and incidence studies have not been reliably done. Cocaine is at present a very common drug of abuse across social classes. The dopamine agonist drugs are usually prescribed for patients for Parkinson's disease, and the bronchodilators for those with a history of asthma.

### Clinical History

Paranoid patients are difficult to interview and are not always forthcoming. Many, however, will answer questions put directly concerning drug usage. The amphetamine abuse history should be elicited from several perspectives, i.e., using a variety of synonyms such as "uppers," "speed," and "black beauties," in addition to "amphetamines." Alcohol consumption, as ever, should be detailed.

## Psychotropic Drug Interaction

Monoamine Oxidase (MAO) Inhibitors. Currently available MAOs inhibit both MAO-A and MAO-B. They are contraindicated for patients taking the drugs discussed in this section. When MAO-B selective inhibitors become available for clinical use, they may be appropriate.

Antipsychotic Drugs. Generally safe.

Cyclic Antidepressants. Because of additive potentiation of catecholaminergic transmission, these drugs should be used with some caution. Patients taking dopamine agonists plus a tricyclic antidepressant may be at greater risk for side effects such as tremor, tachycardia, cardiac arrhythmia, and agitation. Such drugs may be prescribed when appropriate, however.

## Mental Status Examination

Arousal. As always, examine for evidence of delirium (i.e., orientation, serial digit repetition, set-changing tasks requiring sustained attention). If evidence of delirium is present, the toxic differential diagnosis list may be much broader than described here.

Thought Content. As discussed above, paranoid delusions and hallucinations may not be clinically distinguishable from those seen in the schizophreniform disorders. Demographic features of the patients or physical examination findings may be necessary to raise the index of suspicion.

## General Medical Examination

Vital Signs. Tachycardia? Systolic hypertension? Postural hypotension?

Skin. Diaphoresis? Spider angiomata in alcoholism.

GI. Hepatomegaly? Stool guaiac positive?

Skin. Needle tracks for drug injections?

## Neurological Examination

Cranial Nerves. Nystagmus on lateral gaze? Although saccadic pursuits have been reported among schizophrenics, coarse or sustained gaze nystagmus is very suspicious for drug or toxin involvement. Pupils are relatively dilated but reactive in people taking sympathetic agonists (they tend to be dilated in schizophrenia as well, however). Abnormal pupils may be seen in chronic alcoholism—elliptical or poorly reactive small pupils (Argyll Robertson pupils). Isolated extraocular muscle palsies such as lateral rectus paralysis may be seen in Wernicke's syndrome.

## Motor Systems

**Tremor.** Action or postural tremor may be seen either in drug intoxication or in withdrawal states. Adrenergic agonists may induce a fine postural tremor of extended hands.

**Movements.** Amphetamine intoxication may produce stereotypical movements or posturing not commonly seen in noncatatonic schizophrenia. The same is true for dopamine agonists. Typically, these movements appear choreiform, involving face or extremities. They may be subtle, and patients often attempt to "cover" them with purposive movements superimposed.

**Cerebellar Function.** Finger-to-nose, heel-to-shin, and gait ataxia should be tested. Depending on the clinical context, abnormalities on these tests may be evidence for intoxication of withdrawal. In general, no focal findings or left/right asymmetries should be in evidence.

## Reflexes

Reflexes may be hyperreflexic, even to the point of ankle clonus in young people, especially young women. Without asymmetry, these signs are a warning, but are not specific. Sustained clonus is unacceptable for the diagnosis of schizophrenia, as are Babinski signs. Asymmetry of reflexes should not be seen either in the schizophreniform psychoses or in toxic conditions.

## Laboratory and Imaging

Radiologic imaging techniques are generally of no value in this situation.

**Amphetamines.** Urinary aliquot, spot sample, can be sent for toxic screen. Trace amounts may remain present in urine up to 7 days after last drug dosage.

**Alcohol.** Serum assay $> 0.3\%$ is evidence of intoxication. Liver function tests may be elevated (ALT, AST, GGTP), or amylase in various drug abusers.

Left hemisphere ⟷ Primary delusions
(esp. temporal lobe)
Diencephalon ⟷ Auditory hallucination
(ventricle III)
Brainstem ⟷ Thought disorder

**Figure 8.5.** Crude anatomic–clinical correlations in paranoia.

Bronchodilators. Theophylline levels may be measured in serum (10.0–20.0 mg/liter or 55–110 mole/liter therapeutic).

# TUMOR, STROKE, AND TRAUMA

## Paranoia Associated with Focal Disease of the CNS

We are combining these three etiologies in this section, because each represents a type of *focal* disease of the nervous system. Such focal CNS disease is not commonly involved in the generation of paranoid syndromes, and when it is, the pathophysiology is usually obvious.

There are a number of clinical reports linking focal disease of the nervous system with paranoia. Davison and Bagley (1969) have provided a useful overview of such reports. In reviewing autopsy series of more or less unselected psychiatric inpatients performed earlier in this century, an increased prevalence of unsuspected brain tumors is found (1.7–11.2% *vs.* 1.0–1.5% expected). Few if any useful clinical correlations emerged from these older series, however. When one proceeds in the "opposite direction," looking at "schizophrenia-like" psychoses in large series of brain tumor patients, prevalence rates from 0.2% to 3.5% are found. This is possibly higher than expected, although proper comparison groups are difficult to define. Again, no particular clinical psychotic pattern emerges from such studies. After reviewing this evidence, Davison and Bagley suggested the correlations shown in Fig. 8.5, but we have not found such a schema to be of much use in our clinical practice.

Benson and Geschwind (1973) have made the clinical observation of an association between Wernicke's aphasia (posterior region, superior temporal gyrus, left hemisphere) and paranoid behavior. Dr. Geschwind told us in a discussion prior to his death that he thought such people with Wernicke's aphasia presented the best neurologic model for paranoid psychoses, but they were difficult to study effectively because of the language block. His hypotheses in this matter await confirmation by future clinical researchers.

There are also reports of paranoid symptomatology emerging after closed-head trauma of varying degrees (Thompson, 1970). We have seen fully developed paranoid psychoses emerge during the recovery phase of relatively severe closed-head injury. In our experience, this has usually occurred during the amnestic period of the recovery process, and patients had no later recollection of the psychosis.

## Checkpoints—Focal Neurologic Lesions and Paranoia

### Demographics

Too much can be said concerning demographics of stroke, tumor, and trauma, and too little can be said concerning their associations with paranoia to justify discussion here.

### Psychotropic Drug Interactions

Pharmacotherapy of stroke, tumor, and trauma remains relatively nonspecific at this time and does not provide the occasion for important drug interactions with psychotropics.

### Clinical History

The clinical history and the neurologic examination are the checkpoints that are useful in screening for the occasional focal CNS disease/paranoia patient. Age of onset has not generally provided an important clinical guide on our experience, since the "psychiatric" paranoid syndromes may occur throughout the life-span. One must always take caution with regard to stroke when patients are in their sixth decade or older. One important quality of the history concerns rapidity of onset of symptoms. Typically, the psychiatric syndromes have a prodrome over days to weeks when a careful history is elicited from another observer, such as a family member, whereas the "medical" paranoias have a more abrupt onset. Psychosocial stressors are dangerous clues diagnostically, since so many patients with medical–neurologic disease describe them.

---

*Clinical Rule 8.5:* Patients state that psychosocial stressors precede medical and neurological disease as often as psychiatric disease.

---

Tumor patients typically have a prodrome of symptoms that precede overt neurologic signs. There may be headaches, personality alterations, visual changes.

Primary brain tumor patients in early- or middle-adult life may be free of other medical disease. Older patients with metastatic brain tumors may have a history of primary malignancy elsewhere or complaints that might indicate systemic malignancy, such as weight loss, cough or hemoptysis, skin lesions, and others. The most important feature of the clinical history for stroke and trauma is the suddenness of onset. Some stroke processes may "stutter" over hours to days, but both of these processes more commonly strike "like a lightning bolt." Stroke under age 40 is relatively rare and is usually caused by processes other than atherosclerosis. Patients at risk for stroke are those with previously identified hypertension, atherosclerotic vascular disease, and cardiac disease such as arrhythmias (particularly atrial fibrillation) or valvular disease.

## Mental Status Examination

The most worrisome mental status distinction in this area concerns the differentiation of aphasic, usually stroke-related paranoid behavior from "psychiatric" paranoid behavior. Many patients with a posterior or Wernicke's aphasia demonstrate relatively few neurologic signs outside their mental status abnormalities. Features that may help to distinguish these patients from a very disorganized psychotic patient include the following:

1. Both types of patients produce neologisms, but the aphasic patients demonstrate more random, nonrepetitive *paraphasias*. Paraphasias may be literal (substituting a senseless phoneme) or verbal (substituting a senseless word within a language train).
2. Fluent aphasic patients usually do not comprehend language, as opposed to even the most disorganized psychotic patient, who usually shows at least fleeting language comprehension.
3. The aphasic patient may demonstrate a "sincerity of contact," as if he assumes the listener to understand him.

## General Medical Examination

For patients with metastatic tumor and stroke, there are often systemic clues to the underlying pathophysiology. One should remember that most strokes are due to emboli, and most emboli come either from the heart or from the carotid arteries in the neck. The tumor types most likely to metastatize to CNS include lung, breast, renal cell, and melanoma.

Chest. Is there a cough? Areas of focal wheezing? Areas of decreased breath sounds?

Cardiac. Hypertension? Arrhythmia? Left sternal border systolic murmur, which might suggest mitral valve disease? Are there bruits along the carotid arteries in the neck? Xanthomas along Achilles' tendons?

Skin. Melanomas typically have poorly defined borders and multiple coloration. Common areas to look for such lesions include sun-exposed areas and palmar surfaces.

GI. Careful abdominal examination including stool guaiac may be indicated, but GI tumors do not commonly metastatize to brain.

## Neurological Examination

Cranial Nerves. Papilledema? Field deficits to target confrontation?

Sensory. Strokes involving Wernicke's area almost always involve sensory or sensory-association cortex as well. Pinprick may not be so well perceived on the right side of the body. Although the patient may not be able to verbalize this, there may be observable differences in his response to alternating simulation on left and right sides.

Motor. In both stroke and tumor, the basic principles apply. One looks for evidence of subtle asymmetry or clumsiness. Is there a pronator drift? Is there circumduction of one leg?

Reflex. Again, the search for asymmetry or for pathological reflexes continues. After trauma, reflexes may be diffusely and symmetrically brisk, sometimes with bilateral pathologic reflexes such as Babinski signs.

## Laboratory and Imaging

For tumor, stroke, and trauma, the head CT scan remains the single most important technologic tool. It should not be ordered, however, unless there is some clinical evidence from the history or examination that is supportive of the diagnosis of a CNS structural lesion. Paranoid psychosis by itself is insufficient. Some other principles concerning the use of CT scans in these syndromes may increase yield and safety. Strokes, uncomplicated by hemorrhage, may not show up on a CT scan during the first 72 hr after the event. If one's suspicion for stroke is only low to moderate, waiting 3 days will increase the yield. The intravenous injection of ionized contrast agents with the CT scan should be considered but should not done in every case. In recent stroke, there may be some risk for injury of brain tissue from extravasation of contrast material into injured tissues. And more than 90% of all tumors will be identified by an uncontrasted scan. In addition, the contrast injection subjects the patient to the small but real risk of serious allergic response or renal compromise. We must refer the reader to our basic rule concerning contrasted CT scans:

---

*Clinical Rule 8.6:* Do not inject contrast material prior to CT scans unless looking for ateriovenous malformations or tumors. And for tumors, do the uncontrasted scan first.

---

## DEGENERATIVE DISEASES AND PARANOIA

A 76-year-old woman is brought to the hospital under mental hygiene assist after a "low-speed chase" across town in her automobile, during which she violated most known traffic rules. She is a retired school teacher and a spinster. She has been described as "a loner" and "humorless" all her life, which qualities have deepened toward eccentricity since her retirement. On interview, she is guarded but clearly paranoid, refusing to speak at any length with the interviewer "because you work for *them*!"

The central issue in the evaluation and treatment of late-life paranoid psychoses is whether any of them are "psychiatric" disorders in the sense or their occurring independently of active medical or neurologic disease. When Sir Martin Roth used the term "paraphrenia" in 1955, he took the position that schizophrenia could begin during the seventh or eighth decade, just as during earlier phases of the life cycle (Roth, 1955). He felt that this group of "paraphrenic" patients was predominantly female and invariably paranoid in clinical presentation, typically with a history of lifelong schizoid personality features. He stated that dementia was not a clinical feature. In a recent, broad view of the topic, Bridge and Wyatt (1980) point out the relative paucity of clinical research on paraphrenia. Some authors report several clinical subtypes of paraphrenia; others emphasize the importance of sensory deprivation as an etiologic factor; still others have reported positive family histories for schizophrenialike disorders. Careful studies of cognition in these patients are not available. The possibility remains that many have degenerative neurologic diseases. Prospective studies are needed to settle these questions.

Most of the neurodegenerative diseases may demonstrate paranoid psychotic features at various times in their course. We have seen such features among patients with Alzheimer's disease when cognitive decline was relatively early (and we suspect that some Alzheimer's patients are hidden within the paraphrenia patients). Paranoid psychotic features among Parkinson's disease (PD) patients are most often attributable to long-term dopaminergic pharmacotherapy, but such features were described among PD patients during the predrug era (Sweet *et al.*, 1976). Unlike the depressive symptoms associated with

PD, these psychotic features tend to occur later in the disease course, when differential confusion with psychiatric diseases is less likely. Among younger patients with paranoid psychoses, Huntington's disease (HD) may be considered (Caine and Shoulson, 1983). Despite the genetic unity of this disease, a variety of psychopathologic syndromes may be seen early in its course. Schizophrenia is probably the most common misdiagnosis in early HD, with paranoid delusions and auditory hallucinations occurring with some frequency. These patients almost always have some abnormal movements as well as some cognitive loss by the time of onset of psychopathology. Sleep-onset visual or auditory hallucinosis may also be reported by patients with narcolepsy (Davison and Bagley, 1969). These are usually time-circumscribed phenomena but occasionally may be described as longer-lived.

## Checkpoints—Degenerative Diseases and Paranoia

### Demographics

Paraphrenia is a disorder of the seventh and eighth decades. Alzheimer's disease starts to become reasonably common during these decades as well, although it can occur as early as the 40s. Huntington's disease, although determined by a single gene, demonstrates variable onset through early- and mid-adult life. Idiopathic Parkinson's disease demonstrates peak incidence through the fifth, sixth, and seventh decades.

### Clinical History

The degenerative diseases typically demonstrate a prodrome of vague symptomatology for months (sometimes years) prior to onset of clearly definable symptoms. Of course, the psychiatric paranoid disorders may be similar in terms of such a prodrome. A few key clinical features that we check when degenerative diseases come to mind are the following.

Alzheimer's Disease. Is there a history of wandering, or getting lost while driving? Has there been unusual or new confusion in the face of stress or novelty, including an exaggerated response to medications? Has there been a personality change? Sleep disturbance? Has the patient become forgetful? Is there a family history for dementia? Any one of these features in the clinical history may indicate a red flag concerning the early stages of a cerebral degenerative disease.

Huntington's Disease. First of all, a positive family history is a prerequisite for diagnosis of this autosomal-dominant disease. Sometimes people are adopted, however, and sometimes the clinical histories are suppressed. One should always pause for a long time, however, before diagnosing an isolated case of Huntington's disease. We prefer questions such as "Was there anyone who was odd or strange in the family?" Anyone who was in a state mental hospital? Anyone who died in a long-term care hospital? In the individual clinical history, cognitive changes are usually present but subtle by the time of onset of a behavioral syndrome. Movements are usually present early, or the disease is not considered.

---

*Clinical Rule 8.7:* Where there are no movements, there is no Huntington's disease.

---

Parkinson's Disease. PD is not familial, or at least not very familial. Some useful clinical features to ask about in taking the clinical history include new muscle cramps, aches, and pains about shoulders, neck, and hip girdle musculature. "Slowness" of movements and of thought process may be noticed by the patient or by family. Depression or depressionlike symptoms are common during and preceding clinical onset of PD.

## Psychotropic Drug Interactions

An exaggerated delirious response to reasonable dosage of any psychoactive medication may sometimes provide a clue to an underlying degenerative disorder. In our experience, this is especially true for Alzheimer's disease.

PD patients have deterioration in central catecholamine systems, which impair cardiovascular reflexes, including physiologic responses to postural hypotension. Most antidepressants and the low-potency antipsychotics may produce exaggerated difficulties with postural hypotension in these patients.

Most PD patients are taking dopamine agonists of one sort or another and cannot take mixed monoamine oxidase inhibitors (which includes all currently available for psychiatric use). They may be given selective MAO-B inhibitors when these drugs become available, although their psychotropic utility is not yet clear.

## Mental Status Examination

Alzheimer's Disease. Check verbal memory, visual memory, visuospatial navigation, and orientation. Language—specifically, listen for early paraphasias, or comprehension errors.

Huntington's Disease. Check verbal memory and information processing, such as spontaneous word list generation.

Parkinson's Disease. Check information processing. Spontaneous word list generation may be impaired, and speed of thought and responses may be slowed.

## General Medical Examination

Alzheimer's Disease. Nonspecific.

Parkinson's Disease. Facial seborrhea, postural hypotension, and impaired autonomic reflexes such as bradycardia to valsalva maneuver.

Huntington's Disease. Nonspecific.

## Neurologic Examination

Alzheimer's Disease. Cranial nerves—normal; sensory—normal or inconsistent; motor—(+) paratonia, gait, coordination, strength generally nil; reflexes—tendon reflexes normal. Disinhibition reflexes such as snout, grasp, nuchocephalic, and paratonia are typically present.

Parkinson's Disease. Cranial nerves—limited up-gaze and in some PD variants limitation of down-gaze; sensory—normal; motor—increased tone of lead pipe quality. Cogwheeling may be superimposed with slowness of initiating movements and truncal ataxia on turns during ambulation.

Huntington's Disease. Abnormal movements usually choreiform, sometimes athetoid or dystonic.

## Laboratory and Imaging

Alzheimer's Disease. Laboratory tests helpful only to "rule out" other diseases. CT or MR scans may demonstrate atrophy—which is confirmatory but not specific.

Parkinson's Disease. Except for stroke-related or toxin-related parkinsonian syndromes, diagnosis remains clinical.

Huntington's Disease. CT may show atrophy of caudate heads but may not be present early in disease course.

## PARANOIA IN INFECTION AND ENDOCRINE DISTURBANCE

Although there are reports in the older literature of paranoid symptomatology occurring during the course of various CNS infections (Davison and Bagley, 1969), the intercurrent evidence of systemic illness is usually sufficient to avoid serious diagnostic difficulties in most bacterial, fungal, and protozoan infections of the CNS. Psychosis with paranoid features may, however, occur during the course of infection with the human immune deficiency virus (HIV) in the relative absence of systemic signs (Rundell *et al.*, 1986; Halevie-Goldman *et al.*, 1987). At the present time, such patients are likely to be members of high-risk groups (homosexuals, IV drug abusers, multiple-transfusion recipients) and to demonstrate anti-HIV antibodies in serum. The CSF is likely to be abnormal in such patients, as is the MR scan of the head.

With regard to endocrine disturbance and psychosis, there is no evidence for a high degree of association. There are reports of paranoid psychoses appearing in the context of Addison's disease (Gorman and Wortis, 1977), but this is rare. There are also reports of paranoid psychoses appearing during the course of myxedema (Logothetis, 1963), and we have observed paranoid symptoms to emerge during the early stages of the treatment of hypothyroidism with thyroxine. Affective disturbances are more common in this condition.

## REFERENCES

Anderson, W. H. Differential diagnosis of acute psychosis. In Manschreck, T. C. (ed.): *Psychiatric Medicine Update, Massachusetts General Hospital Reviews for Physicians.* New York: Elsevier, 1979; pp. 103–108.

Arana, G. W., Goff, D. C., Friedman, H., Ornsteen, M., Greenblatt, D. J., Black, B., and Shader, R. I. Does carbamozepine-induced reduction of plasma haloperidol levels worsen psychotic symptoms? *Am. J. Psychiatry*, 1986, **143,** 650–651.

Bell, D. S. Comparison of amphetamine psychosis and schizophrenia. *Br. J. Psychiatry*, 1965, **111,** 701–707.

Benson, D. F. Psychiatric aspects of aphasia. *Br. J. Psychiatry*, 1973, **123,** 555–566.

Benson D. F., and Geschwind, N. Psychiatric conditions associated with focal lesions of the central nervous system. In Arieti S. (ed.): *American Handbook of Psychiatry*. New York: Basic Books, 1973, Chap. 9.

Blumer, D. Temporal lobe epilepsy and its psychiatric significance. In Benson, D. F., and Blumer, D. (eds.): *Psychiatric Aspects of Neurologic Disease*. New York: Grune and Stratton, 1975, pp. 171–198.

Bridge, T. P., and Wyatt, R. J. Paraphenia: Paranoid states of late life. I. European research. II. American research. *J. Am. Geriatr. Soc.*, 1980, **28,** 193–205.

Bridgers, S. L. Epileptiform abnormalities discovered on electroencephalographic screening of psychiatric inpatients. *Arch. Neurol.*, 1987, **44,** 312–316.

Caine, E. D., and Shoulson, I. Psychiatric syndromes in Huntington's disease. *Am. J. Psychiatry*, 1983, **140,** 728–733.

Connell, P. H. *Amphetamine Psychosis*, Maudsley Monograph No. 5. London: Chapman and Hall, 1958.

Currie, S., Heathfield, K. W. G., Henson, R. A., and Scott, D. F. Clinical course and prognosis of temporal lobe epilepsy: A survey of 666 patients. *Brain*, 1971, **94,** 173–190.

Davison, K., and Bagley, D. Schizophrenia-like psychoses associated with organic disorders of the central nervous system. In Herrington, R. N. (ed.): *Current Problems in Neuropsychiatry*. London: Headley Bros., 1969.

Delgado-Escueta, A. V. Epileptogenic paraoxysms: Modern approaches and clinical correlations. *Neurology*, 1979, **29,** 1014–1022.

*Diagnostic and Statistical Manual of Mental Disorders*, 3d ed., revised. Washington, DC: American Psychiatric Association, 1987.

Dongier, S. Statistical study of clinical and electroencephalographic manifestations of 536 psychotic episodes occurring in 516 epileptics between clinical seizures. *Epilepsia*, 1959/1960, **1,** 117–142.

Fraser, A. A., and Ingram, I. M. Lorazepam dependence and chronic psychosis. *Br. J. Psychiatry*, 1985, **147,** 211 (letter).

Gastaut, H., Gastaut, J. L., Silva, G. E. G., and Sanchez, G. R. F. Relative frequency of different types of epilepsy: A study employing the classification of the International League against Epilepsy. *Epilepsia*, 1975, **16,** 457–461.

Gay, P. E., and Madsen, J. A. Interaction between phenobarbital and thioridazine. *Neurology (NY)*, 1983, **33,** 1631–1632.

Goldensohn, E. S., and Gold, A. P. Prolonged behavioral disturbances as ictal phenomena. *Neurology (NY)*, 1960, **10,** 1–9.

Gorman, W. F., and Wortis, S. B. Psychosis in Addison's disease. *Dis. Nerv. Syst.*, 1947, **8,** 267–271.

Hackett, T. P. Alcoholism: Acute and chronic states. In Hackett, T. P., and Cassem, N. H. (eds.): *Massachusetts General Hospital Handbook of General Hospital Psychiatry*, St. Louis: C. V. Mosby, 1978, pp. 15–28.

Halevie-Goldman, B. D., Potkin, S. G., and Poyourow, P. AIDS-related complex presenting as psychosis. *Am. J. Psychiatry*, 1987, **144,** 964 (letter).

Hermann, B. P., Dikmen, S., Schwartz, M. S., and Karnes, W. E. Interictal psychopathology in patients with ictal fear: A quantitative investigation. *Neurology (NY)*, 1982, **32,** 7–11.

Hughes, J. R., and Wilson, W. P. (eds.). *EEG and Evoked Potentials in Psychiatry and Behavioral Neurology*. Woburn, MA: Butterworth, 1983.

Kane, F. J., and Florenzano R. Psychosis accompanying use of bronchodilator compound. *JAMA*, 1971, **215,** 2116 (letter).

Landolt, H. Some clinical electroencephalographic correlations in epileptic psychoses (twilight states). *Electroencephalogr. Clin. Neurophysiol.*, 1953, **5,** 121.

Levin, M. Bromide psychosis: Four varieties. *Am. J. Psychiatry*, 1948, **104,** 798–800.

Linnoila, M., Viukari, M., Vaisanen, K., and Auvinen, J. Effect on anticonvulsants on plasma haloperidol and thioridazine levels. *Am. J. Psychiatry*, 1980, **137,** 819–821.

Logothetis, J. Psychotic between as the initial indicator of adult myxedema. *J. Nerv. Ment. Dis.*, 1963, **136,** 516–568.

Logothetis, J. Spontaneous epileptic seizures and electroencephalographic changes in the course of phenothiazine therapy. *Neurology*, 1967, **17,** 869–877.

McKenna, P. J., Kane, J. M., and Parrish, K. Psychotic syndromes in epilepsy. *Am. J. Psychiatry*, 1985, **142,** 895–904.

Medical Letter. *Med. Lett. Drugs Ther*, 1986, **28,** 69–72.

Mendez, M. F., Cummings, J. L., and Benson, D. F. Epilepsy: Psychiatric aspects and use of psychotropics. *Psychosomatics*, 1984, **25,** 883–894.

*Mental Disorders: Glossary and Guide to Their Classification in Accordance with the Ninth Revision of the International Classification of Diseases.* Geneva: World Health Organization, 1978.

Neufeld, M. Y., Cohn, D. F., and Korczyn, A. D. Sphenoidal EEG recording in complex partial seizures. *Neurology*, 1986, **36** (Suppl. 1), 87 (abstract).

Oliver, A. P., Luchins, D. J., and Wyatt, R. J. Neuroleptic-induced seizures: An *in vitro* technique for assessing relative risk. *Arch. Gen. Psychiatry*, 1982, **39,** 206–209.

Pakalnis, A., Drake, M. E., John, K., and Kellum, J. B. Forced normalization: Acute psychosis after seizure control in seven patients. *Arch. Neurol.*, 1987, **44,** 289–292.

Pampiglione, G., and Kerridge, J. EEG abnormalities from the temporal lobe studied with sphenoidal electrodes. *J. Neurol. Neurosurg. Psychiatr.*, 1956, **19,** 117–129.

Perez, M. M., and Trimble, M. R. Epileptic psychosis—diagnostic comparison with process schizophrenia. *Br. J. Psychiatry*, 1980, **137,** 245–249.

Pincus, J. H., and Tucker, G. J. Seizures Disorders. In Pincus, J. H. and Tucker, G. J. (eds.): *Behavioral Neurology*, 3d ed. New York: Oxford University Press, 1985, pp. 3–57.

Ramani, V., Loewenson, R. B., and Torres, F. The limited usefulness of nasopharyngeal EEG recording in psychiatric patients. *Am. J. Psychiatry*, 1985, **142,** 1099–1100.

Roberts, K., and Vass, N. Schneiderian first-rank symptoms caused by benzodiazepine withdrawal. *Br. J. Psychiatry*, 1986, **148,** 593–594.

Roth, M. The natural history of mental disorder in old age. *J. Ment. Sci*, 1955, **101,** 281–301.

Rovit, R. L., Gloor, P., and Rasmussen, T. Sphenoidal electrodes in the electrographic study of patients with temporal lobe epilepsy: An evaluation. *J. Neurosurg.*, 1961, **18,** 151–158.

Rundell, J. R., Wise, M. G., and Ursano, R. J. Three cases of AIDS-related psychiatric disorders. *Am. J. Psychiatry*, 1986, **143,** 777–778.

Sabot, L. M., Gross, M. M., and Halpert, E. A study of acute alcoholic psychoses in women. *Br. J. Addict.*, 1968, **63,** 29–49.

Shader, R. I. *Psychiatric Complications of Medical Drugs.* New York: Raven Press, 1972.

Sherwin, I., Peron-Magnan, P., Bancaud, J., Bonis, A., and Talairach, J. Prevalence of psychosis in epilepsy as a function of the laterality of the epileptogenic lesion. *Arch. Neurol.*, 1982, **39,** 621–625.

Simpson, J. A. The clinical neurology of temporal lobe disorders. In Herrington, R. N. (ed.): *Current Problems in Neuropsychiatry. Br. J. Psychiatry*, Special Publication No. 4, 1969, pp. 42–48.

Slater, E. The schizophrenia-like illnesses of epilepsy. In Herrington, R. N. (ed.): *Current Problems in Neuropsychiatry.* London: Headley Bros., 1969, pp. 77–81.

Slater, E., Beard, A. W., and Glitheroe, E. The schizophrenia-like psychoses of epilepsy. *Br. J. Psychiatry*, 1963, **109,** 95–105.

Special Report of International Workshop on Aggression and Epilepsy. *N. Engl. J. Med.*, 1981, **305,** 711–716.

Stephens, D. A. Psychotoxic effects of benzhexol hydrochloride (Artane). *Br. J. Psychiatry*, 1967, **113,** 213–218.

Stevens, J. R. Psychiatric implications of psychomotor epilepsy *Arch. Gen. Psychiatry*, 1966, **14,** 461–471.

Stevens, J. R., and Herman, B. P. Temporal lobe epilepsy, psychopathology and violence: The state of the evidence. *Neurology*, 1981, **31,** 1127–1132.

Stoudemire, A., Nelson, A., and Houpt, J. L. Interictal schizophrenia-like psychoses in temporal lobe epilepsy. *Psychosomatics*, 1983, **24,** 331–339.

Sweet, R. D., McDowell, F. H., Feigenson, J. S., Loranger, A. W., and Goodell, H. Mental symptoms in Parkinson's disease during chronic treatment with levodopa. *Neurology (NY)*, 1976, **26,** 305–310.

Talbott, J. A., and Teague, J. W. Marijuana psychosis: Acute toxic psychosis associated with the use of *Cannabis* derivatives. *JAMA*, 1969, **210,** 299–302.

Taneli, B., Ozaskinli, S., Kirli, S., Erden, G., and Bura, I. Bromocriptine-induced schizophrenic syndrome. *Am. J. Psychiatry*, 1986, **143,** 935 (letter).

Thompson, G. N. Cerebral lesions simulating schizophrenia: Three case reports. *Biol. Psychiatry*, 1970, **2,** 59–64.

Toone, B. K., Garralda, M. E., and Ron, M. A. The psychoses of epilepsy and the functional psychoses: A clinical and phenomenological comparison. *Br. J. Psychiatry*, 1982, **141,** 256–261.

Trimble, M. R. Psychiatric and psychological aspects of epilepsy. In Porter, R. J., and Morselli, P. L. (eds.): *Epilepsies*, Vol. 5. Kent, U.K.: Butterworths, 1984, pp. 325–355.

Trimble, M. R. The psychoses of epilepsy and their treatment. In Trimble, M. R. (ed.): *The Psychopharmacology of Epilepsy*. Chichester, U.K.: John Wiley and Sons, 1985, pp. 83–94.

Victor, M., and Hope, J. M. The phenomenon of auditory hallucinations in chronic alcoholism. A critical evaluation of the status of alcoholic hallucinosis. *J. Nerv. Ment. Dis*, 1958, **126,** 451–481.

Whitehouse, A. M., and Duncan, J. M. Ephedrine psychosis rediscovered. *Br. J. Psychiatry*, 1987, **150,** 258–261.

Williams, D. The structure of emotions reflected in epileptic experiences. *Brain*, 1956, **79,** 28–67.

Woodbury, D. M., Penry, J. K., and Pippenger, C. E. *Antiepileptic Drugs*, 2d ed. New York: Raven Press, 1982, pp. 234–336.

# 9

# Nonparanoid Psychosis

### DSM-III-R Disorders

*Alcoholic Hallucinosis.* An organic hallucinosis in which vivid and persistent hallucinations develop shortly after cessation of or reduction in alcohol ingestion by a person who apparently has alcohol dependence.

*Amphetamine Delusional Disorder*

*Cannabis Delusional Disorder*

*Cocaine Delusional Disorder*

*Hallucinogen Hallucinosis and Delusional Disorder*

*Phencyclidine Delusional Disorder*

*Schizophrenia, Catatonic Type.* A type of schizophrenia in which the clinical picture is dominated by any of the following:

1. Catatonic stupor
2. Catatonic negativism
3. Catatonic rigidity
4. Catatonic excitement
5. Catatonic posturing

*Schizophrenia, Disorganized Type.* A type of schizophrenia in which the following criteria are met:

1. Incoherence, marked loosening of associations, or grossly disorganized behavior
2. Flat or grossly inappropriate affect

*Schizophrenia, Undifferentiated Type.* A type of schizophrenia in which there are prominent delusions, hallucinations, incoherence, or grossly disorganized behavior.

*Schizophrenia, Residual Type.* A type of schizophrenia in which there are:

1. Absence of prominent delusions, hallucinations, incoherence, or grossly disorganized behavior.
2. Continuing evidence of the disturbance, as indicated by two or more residual symptoms.

*Brief Reactive Psychosis.* The sudden onset of psychotic symptoms of at least a few hours' but no more than 1 month's duration, with eventual full return to premorbid level of functioning.

*Schizophreniform Disorder.* A disorder identical with schizophrenia except that the duration, including prodromal, active, and residual phases, is less than 6 months.

*Induced Psychotic Disorder.* The essential feature of this disorder is a delusional system that develops in a second person as a result of a close relationship with another person who already has a psychotic disorder with prominent delusions.

*Psychotic Disorder Not Otherwise Specified (Atypical Psychosis).* Disorders in which there are psychotic symptoms (delusions, hallucinations, incoherence, marked loosening of associations, catatonic excitement or stupor, or grossly disorganized behavior) that do not meet the criteria for any other nonorganic psychotic disorder.

**ICD-9 Disorders**

*Schizophrenia, Simple Type.* A psychosis in which there is insidious development of oddities of conduct, inability to meet the demands of society, and decline in total performance. Delusions and hallucinations are not in evidence and the condition is less obviously psychotic than are the hebephrenic, catatonic, and paranoid types of schizophrenia. With increasing social impoverishment, vagrancy may ensue and the patient becomes self-absorbed, idle, and aimless.

*Schizophrenia, Hebephrenic Type.* A form of schizophrenia in which affective changes are prominent, delusions and hallucinations fleeting and unpredictable, and mannerisms common. The mood is shallow and inappropriate accompanied by giggling or self-satisfied, self-absorbed smiling, or by a lofty manner, grimaces, mannerisms, pranks, hypochondriacal complaints, and reiterated phrases. Thought is disorganized. There is a tendency to remain solitary, and behavior seems empty of purpose and feeling.

*Schizophrenia, Catatonic Type.* Includes as an essential feature prominent psychomotor disturbances often alternating between extremes such as hyperkinesis and stupor, or automatic obedience and negativism. Constrained attitudes may be maintained for long periods: if the patient's limbs are put in some unnatural position they may be held there for some time after the external force has been removed. Severe excitement may be a striking feature of the condition. Depressive or hypomanic concomitants may be present.

*Acute Schizophrenic Episode.* Schizophrenic disorders, other than those listed above, in which there is a dreamlike state with slight clouding of consciousness and perplexity. External things, people and events may become charged with personal significance for the patient. There may be ideas of reference and emotional turmoil. In many such cases remission occurs within a few weeks or months, even without treatment.

One can see from reviewing this somewhat long and varied list of psychiatric diagnoses that we will be discussing a heterogeneous group of disorders in this chapter. At the risk of simplification, the four diagnostic issues that confront the clinician within this category of nonparanoid psychoses are these: (1) catatonic syndromes; (2) psychotic states prominently characterized by disorders of thought process; (3) hallucinations; (4) nonparanoid delusions.

Delusional syndromes are usually attributable to psychiatric disease. Syndromes of increased muscle tone including catatonia, disturbed thought process, and hallucinations, however, must be carefully considered whenever they are newly evaluated. The possibility of intercurrent neurologic or general medical disease is very real among such patients. Opportunities for diagnostic error abound. There are probably two fundamental reasons why this diagnostic evaluation can be so difficult. On the one hand, almost *any* medical or neurologic disease, once it involves the central nervous system, is capable of disrupting thought process, disturbing motor systems, or producing hallucinations. On the other hand, the "psychiatric" nonparanoid psychoses are probably more closely "neurological" in their origins than the other major psychiatric syndromes. We will discuss this issue first.

There have been a number of reports of structural brain abnormalities among schizophrenic patients (Tsai *et al.*, 1983; Nasrallah, *et al.*, 1982; Andreasen *et al.*, 1982a). The abnormalities that have been reported by some investigative groups have included enlargement of third and lateral ventricles, gyral atrophy with sulcal enlargement across cortex, and reversal of the "normal" left occipital enlargement. In addition, there are reports of a variety of histopathologic abnormalities in periventricular, diencephalic, and prefrontal cortical areas of schizophrenic brains (Weinberger *et al.*, 1987). There is evidence that the schizophrenic patients with such structural brain changes by CT scan tend to be those with negative symptoms and signs, such as affective flattening and avolition (Andreasen *et al.*, 1982b). They may be more difficult to treat with standard antipsychotic medication (Weinberger *et al.*, 1980). And there is evidence that these patients demonstrate a variety of cognitive impairments including impaired verbal IQ scores on the Wechsler Adult Intelligence Scale, and of language and arithmetic skills on the Luria-Nebraska Battery (Luchins *et al.*, 1982; Golden *et al.*, 1980).

It is of further interest for this book that patients with severe and chronic schizophrenia also demonstrate abnormalities on their neurological examinations. Hypertonicity, flexion posturing, choreiform and stereotypical movements, and saccadic visual pursuits have all been described (Weinreb, 1983; Rogers, 1985). The so-called "soft" or nonlocalizing signs are also found more often among schizophrenic patients in general than among other psychiatric patients (Rochford *et al.*, 1970). When such examinations are confined to the various schizophrenic subtypes, the "process" schizophrenic patients demon-

**Table 9.1**
Neurologic Soft Signs Helpful in Discriminating Process from Nonprocess Schizophrenia

| | |
|---|---|
| Dysdiadochokinesia | Finger–thumb mirror movements |
| Face–hand test | Awkward fine finger movements |
| Agraphesthesia | Awkward hopping on one foot |

strate more abnormal neurologic signs than the others (Quitken *et al.*, 1976). Those neurologic signs that have proved discriminating are presented in Table 9.1.

It is difficult to be sure of the correct interpretation of such data. They may indicate that nonparanoid schizophrenia is a particularly malignant mental disease, capable of affecting CNS motor systems as well as those systems involved in the mental status. Or they may indicate that such patients are a heterogeneous group, with subgroups of congenitally or otherwise brain-damaged persons included. Certainly these data indicate that abnormal findings on neurologic examination as well as abnormal performance on cognitive tests will not be as helpful diagnostically, since they may be commonly found among patients with the psychiatric disorders under diagnostic consideration. Perhaps more than any other major diagnostic area, clinical experience will prove the best arbiter for these nonparanoid psychoses.

Delirium, hallucinations, and catatonic syndromes present the psychiatric clinician with a dilemma similar to that posed by nonparanoid schizophrenia. Whereas some nonparanoid schizophrenic patients demonstrate abnormal cognition, neurologic findings, and abnormal neuroimaging studies, delirious or catatonic patients demonstrate disturbances of thought, affect, and perception that are neuropathologically based. "Delirium" refers to an abnormal mental status that is usually produced by toxic or metabolic interference with neuronal function. The confused, fluctuating, thought-disordered picture it presents, however, more closely resembles the nonparanoid psychoses than any other psychiatric syndrome. And when advanced to a sufficient degree, *any* neurologic or medical disease may produce a delirious picture. Similarly, catatonic states are reasonably common among neurologic diseases but are widely equated in the "group preconscious" of clinicians with catatonic schizophrenia. "Hallucination" sounds like a simple enough phenomenon, but on reflection the concept turns out to be difficult to define and heterogeneous. Moreover, it is probably the case that a majority of hallucinations "seen" in clinical practice are attributable to neurologic disease, at least according to some definitions of the term. In view of the central importance of these three types of clinical phenomena within psychiatric diagnosis, we present brief overviews of neurologic considerations relevant to each.

## DELIRIUM

"Delirium" refers to a toxic or metabolic confusional state of variable symptomatology that is often mistaken for psychosis. For reviews of the topic see Engel and Romano (1959) and Lipowski (1967, 1987). On the mental status examination, the essential finding is an impairment of *arousal*. When early or mild, this takes the form of a subtle, fluctuating disturbance in attention focusing and concentration, but as the syndrome becomes more clinically advanced, more global difficulties with alertness may be seen. Occasionally, there are states of paradoxical hyperalertness and agitation, probably analogous to disinhibitory behavior seen in intoxications. This disturbance in attention-regulating and consciousness mechanisms is almost certainly attributable to mild, diffuse impairment of frontal lobe and reticular activating neuronal mechanisms in the brainstem.

When a delirium takes the form primarily of a disturbance of arousal with hypoalertness and increased somnolence, the neurologic term "encephalopathy" is often applied. Fortunately or unfortunately for clinical psychiatrists, in some people a much wider and sometimes florid array of mental status symptomatology may occur. Common findings secondary to the arousal defect but occurring in other mental status functions include disorientation, mild disturbance of thought process ("confusion"), visual illusions or hallucinations, and sometimes delusions. All are worse at night. The reasons why some people appear psychotic during an early metabolic encephalopathy while others merely appear sleepy are unknown. Persons at either end of the life-span (children and the elderly) seem to be more vulnerable than those in the middle. Persons with an underlying dementia or other structural brain disease are also at increased risk. We are far from convinced that individual life histories and psychodynamics are irrelevant. In some of the older literature, the importance of individual premorbid life experience in determining "thresholds" for the onset of delirium as well as for determining symptomatic content was stressed (Ebaugh *et al.*, 1936; Wolff and Curran, 1935), and we suspect that such matters are relevant.

It would be easier for clinical practice if delirium could always be attributed to the presence of a metabolic or pharmacologic neurotoxin. Although this is usually the case, there are two exceptions that are useful to remember. First, we have no doubt that certain psychiatric diseases (mania, schizophrenia) are capable of producing delirious mental states. Relatively little has been written of this recently, but the older literature describes such syndromes quite well, and we have seen them (Hanes, 1912). Second, focal neurologic disease, especially stroke involving the posterior portion of the right cerebral hemisphere in right handers, or stroke involving mesial and inferior temporal lobe structures may cause a "focal neurologic delirium" (Mesulam *et al.*, 1976;

**Table 9.2**
Clinical and Laboratory Features of Delirium

| |
|---|
| Major features (required) |
| Clinical history of acute or subacute onset |
| Mental status examination shows impairment of attention, arousal, or concentration |
| Concurrent neuromedical disease or toxic condition capable of producing encephalopathy |
| At least one abnormal laboratory parameter consistent with clinical impression |
| Minor features (confirmatory) |
| Patient's age at one extreme of life cycle (i.e., childhood or elderly) |
| Nocturnal exacerbation of confusion |
| Visual hallucinations |
| Presence of carphologia |
| Slowing of EEG background rhythm |

Medina *et al.*, 1977). The neurologic findings outside the mental status abnormalities may be quite subtle in such patients and are often confined to visual and cortical sensory abnormalities.

We suggest a clinical approach to the diagnosis of delirium, which is presented in Table 9.2. This outline requires that the patient's medical history be reviewed and mental status examined but also that the laboratory evaluation be scrutinized. An abnormal laboratory parameter capable of explaining the mental picture must be found, and on occasion the psychiatrist may need to participate in the metabolic evaluation to locate such a parameter. The EEG is not usually of help in this diagnostic assessment, since mild background slowing of alpha rhythm, for example, to the nine-cycles-per-second range, may not be known to be abnormal for a given individual. It is most useful in cases where, for some reason, a previous EEG has been performed that can be used for comparison.

When all major criteria listed in Table 9.2 are not present, the clinician who suspects delirium should think again. The clinical picture may still be due to metabolic encephalopathy, but the burden of proof remains with the clinician. Could this be one of the focal neurologic confusional states? Could this be confusion secondary to a psychiatric disease (i.e., mania or schizophrenia)? Could this be an acute psychosis as a defensive response to psychologic or psychosocial events?

## CATATONIA

*Clinical Rule 9.1:* Catatonia is a neurologic sign—not a disease.

The patient was often seen standing in the middle of the corridor, in a stiff posture with his arms pressed against his legs, staring in front of him while he talked as it

> were to the air in a loud voice. . . . He would also gesticulate with his arms or make religious ceremonial movements and other signs, or write in the air. At times during this behavior he assumed very strange postures.
>
> *Kahlbaum, 1874*

"Catatonia" has been used to refer both to a neurologic sign and to a neuropsychiatric syndrome. As a sign, it indicates the finding of non-velocity-dependent increased muscle tone, accompanied by the propensity to maintain passively assumed postures. As a syndrome, the boundaries are hazy, but the term has generally been used to indicate the constellation of catalepsy, negativism, mutism, stereotypy, posturing, muscular rigidity, and verbigeration (Stoudemire, 1982). Agitation and hyperactivity are sometimes included within the syndrome concept. The catatonic syndrome appears in the course of a wide variety of neuromedical diseases (Gelenberg, 1976; Penn *et al.*, 1972; Tippin and Dunner, 1981; Newmann, 1955; Hockaday *et al.*, 1966; Schwab and Barrow, 1964; Woods, 1980). A tabulation of such neuromedical disorders that have been reported in association with all or part of the catatonic syndrome is presented in Table 9.3.

Table 9.3 is more encyclopedic than incisive. Some of the disorders listed are much more likely than others to produce catatonia, and they will be discussed in profile fashion later in this chapter. As in any obsessive list, we have placed the (clinically) most important cause of catatonia last. It is our experi-

**Table 9.3**
Medical and Neurologic Diseases Associated with Catatonia[a]

| |
|---|
| Neurologic disorders |
| Basal ganglion disorders |
| Limbic system and temporal lobe disorders, including limbic encephalitis |
| Diencephalic disorders, including third ventricular hemorrhage and tumor |
| Miscellaneous hemispheric lesions |
| Metabolic conditions |
| Diabetic ketoacidosis |
| Hypercalcemia |
| Pellagra |
| Homocystinuria |
| Hepatic encephalopathy |
| Toxins |
| Organic fluorides |
| Illuminating gases |
| Mescaline |
| Ethanol |
| Phencyclidine (PCP) |
| Neuroleptics |

[a]Reprinted in part from Stoudemire (1982), with permission.

ence that antipsychotic drugs are probably the most common cause of catatonia, at least in our hospital, and that psychiatrists sometimes hesitate to recognize the connection. Severe metabolic derangements involving calcium and frontal lobe brain tumors are also encountered with some frequency. The remaining etiologies on the list are useful for roundsmanship.

Features of the catatonic syndrome may also be seen during the course of the major psychiatric disorders. The list of such psychiatric disorders is also long. When Abrams and Taylor (1976) reviewed the psychiatric diagnoses among 55 consecutive psychiatric inpatients with catatonic signs, they found them distributed across affective disorders, the schizophrenias, "organic" mental syndromes, and reactive psychoses. "Lethal catatonia" as well, a syndrome of fever, confusion, motor driveness, and exhaustion, has been associated with a variety of psychiatric diseases (Mann *et al.*, 1986). Indeed, when chronic schizophrenic patients are examined neurologically, it may be that a majority demonstrate increased tone and postural abnormalities (Rogers, 1985).

## HALLUCINATIONS

It is difficult to make useful general statements about the clinical problem of hallucinations. The range of sensory phenomena that may be subsumed under this concept is so broad that it is matched only by the array of neurophysiologic and psychophysiologic events that may cause them. Perhaps more than any other sign or symptom considered in this book, the diagnostic consideration of hallucinations cannot be separated from the individual clinical context.

Hallucinations may affect any of the five sensory modalities, or they may cross or distort modalities. As an example of the phenomenologic complexity the clinician may face, consider the following range of symptoms which may all be subsumed under hallucinations of the visual system (Table 9.4).

When the clinician thinks about a hallucination from a neurophysiologic perspective, he is forced to consider an entire sensory system, from peripheral receptors through central pathways to sensory cortex and association cortex. In visual hallucinations, for example, pathology anywhere within the retina–optic nerves–optic tracts–optic radiations–occipital lobe–temporal association cortex may be implicated. Generalizations can be made concerning "formed" versus "unformed" hallucinations. Typically, the more complex, multimodality, or "formed" the hallucination, the more likely it is to be referrable to dysfunction of temporal or occipital association cortex. "Unformed" hallucinations are more likely to be attributed to retinal or visual cortex pathology. Only peduncular hallucinosis (vivid, nonstereotypical, colorful imagery that is nonthreatening) may be of good localizing value, and the significant brainstem abnormalities

**Table 9.4**
Hallucinations of the Visual System

| Symptom | Anatomy |
|---|---|
| Formed visual hallucinations | Occipital association cortex. When integrated with sound or true memory of past experience—temporal neocortex. May also be brainstem |
| Unformed visual hallucinations | Occipital cortex (migraine); ocular pathology also possible |
| Eidetic imagery | Unknown |
| Phosphenes (flashes of light) | Ocular; optic tracts; occipital cortex |
| Chromatopsias (abnormal tints) | Occipital association cortex—temporal cortex |
| Metachromatopsia (one color changed to another) | Same as chromatopsia |
| Allesthesia (real object appears displaced) | Temporal lobe |
| Palinopsia (image remains after stimulus is removed) | |
| Metamorphopsia (distortion of shape) | |
| Micropsia/teleopsia (objects appear small and distant) | Temporal lobe |
| Macropsia (objects appear magnified) | Temporal lobe |

that usually accompany this phenomenon make localization from the sensory findings unnecessary (Geller and Bellur, 1987).

We have "seen" all or most of these hallucinations among patients with psychiatric diseases as well, especially among schizophrenics. At the risk of ranging even further afield than usual, we provide one clinical rule with regard to hallucinations before proceeding with our more systematic review of medical and neurologic diseases associated with nonparanoid psychosis.

*Clinical Rule 9.2:* Visual hallucinations in nonschizophrenics are due to occult medical or neurologic disease. Auditory hallucinations in nonepileptic patients are psychiatric. Tactile, olfactory, and gustatory hallucinations are due to medical/neurologic disease.

*Caveat*: Experienced clinicians may override this rule, but only after "seeing" the patient.

Our plan now is to return to our outline of other chapters and to discuss the medical and neurological differential diagnosis of nonparanoid psychotic states. Since we will consider any of the previous three clinical constellations

**Table 9.5**
Neuromedical Syndromes Associated with Nonparanoid Psychosis

| | |
|---|---|
| Metabolic disorders | Drug and toxin |
| Hepatic encephalopathy | Benzodiazepines |
| Wilson's disease | Corticosteroids |
| Deficiency syndromes | Belladonna alkaloids |
| Hypercalcemia | Antiparkinsonian drugs |
| Infection | Hallucinogens |
| CNS—viral | Dopamine-blocking drugs |
| Non-CNS infections | Antiemetics |
| Endocrine | Tumor and trauma |
| Thyrotoxicosis | Epilepsy |
| | Psychomotor status |
| | Stroke |
| | Wernicke's syndrome |
| | Acute confusional strokes |

(catatonic states, disorganized confusional states, and hallucinations) to qualify as "nonparanoid psychosis," we must address a more heterogeneous group of neuromedical diseases. We propose to consider those which, in our experience, have proved to be the most likely, which we have listed in Table 9.5.

## DRUGS AND TOXINS ASSOCIATED WITH NONPARANOID PSYCHOSIS

### Catatonic Syndromes

A 31-year-old woman with multiple sclerosis experienced a manic syndrome while receiving a short course of high-dose corticosteroids. Her neurologist prescribed molindone as therapy for the mania and increased this drug to 30 mg/day. Instead of improving, the patient became disorganized to the point of incoherence. She became incontinent of bowel and bladder. Progressive motor stiffness with abnormal posturing supervened. On mental status examination, she rhythmically repeated a single word, "moban," for hours at a time.

Drugs that act by producing dopamine blockade, such as the antipsychotics and antiemetics that increase GI motility such as metoclopramide, are the most common causes of drug-induced catatonia. Two issues have been raised with regard to such catatonic (and catastrophic) drug reactions. One is that they may simply be "total-body" dystonias. We would disagree with this contention on clinical grounds. Patients with catatonia as a drug side effect may demonstrate true waxy flexibility of muscle tone, as opposed to the rigidity of parkinsonism or the episodic hypertonicity of dystonia. In addition, the other signs of the catatonic syndrome, such as verbigeration in our illustration, are likely to accompany the motor system findings. Another important question is whether these catatonic drug reactions are in fact *forme frustes* of the neuroleptic malignant syndrome (NMS)—the clinical triad of rigidity, autonomic hyperactivity, and mental confusion. We are not so sure about this question. These syndromes do demonstrate considerable clinical overlap, and we would not be surprised if future research links them neuroanatomically or neurophysiologically.

Certain psychoactive drugs of abuse, including phencyclidine and marijuana, are also associated with the clinical finding of catalepsy (Nicholi, 1983). Phencyclidine induces a vestibulocerebellar syndrome at doses that produce mental status alterations, so the neurologic examination may be of help in diagnosis. Findings of particular relevance include nystagmus and an inability to perform the Romberg maneuver. Marijuana typically produces an elevation in heart rate and an elevation in systolic blood pressure, although these findings are not specific. Both drugs produce impairments in attention and concentration on mental status examination. Both may be detected in serum and urine toxicological screens.

There are more anecdotal reports of catatonic syndromes having been produced by such compounds as illuminating gas, fluorides, aspirin, amphetamines, and alcohol (Herman *et al.*, 1942; Schwab and Barrow, 1964). These syndromes must be clinical rarities, however. One can work much more effectively in evaluating catatonic syndromes by briefly considering the four types of drugs discussed above: Can this be secondary to an antipsychotic? Can this be secondary to antinausea medication? Can this be secondary to phencyclidine or marijuana? Can this be secondary to an anti-Parkinson's medication?

## Confusional States

The problem with drug-induced confusional states, which may mimic the disorganized, thought-disordered psychoses, is that there are so many of them. Almost any medication, if taken to an individual's toxic dose, can produce such a mental status picture (Shader, 1972). In Table 9.4 we have listed the categories of drugs including benzodiazepines, corticosteroids, and belladonna alkaloids as particular offenders. No comprehensive list is possible. In our experience, benzodiazepines, especially diazepam and chlordiazepoxide, are very suspicious agents when they appear on the medication list of a psychotic patient, as are all anticholinergic drugs. Certain physical findings are usually present in both classes of agents. Patients on benzodiazepines have nystagmus, and when more intoxicated, cerebellar gait ataxia appears. Patients receiving anticholinergics develop dry mucous membranes, facial flushing, and decreased bowel sounds. The elderly and teenagers may be especially vulnerable to the development of confusional states while taking relatively low doses of these medications (McGucken and Caldwell, 1985), and patients with underlying structural neurologic disease such as Alzheimer's diseases are especially vulnerable (Sunderland *et al.*, 1987).

## Hallucinatory States

Psychotic states characterized by relatively prominent hallucinations are most likely to be produced, in our experience, by two classes of agents: the antiparkinsonian dopamine agonists, and the drugs of abuse that are often categorized together as "hallucinogens." It is not uncommon in clinical practice for hallucinatory experiences to appear in the context of a toxic delirium due to almost any agent. For example, Table 9.6 provides a long list of agents that have been reported to produce such hallucinatory toxic states (Medical Letter, 1986).

For most of the drugs listed in Table 9.6, the hallucinatory states are visual as opposed to auditory, and they occur in the context of a confusional state. Arousal, attention, and concentration are impaired. Appropriate diagnostic suspicion is usually aroused easily. We have been impressed, however, that

**Table 9.6**
Drugs That May Produce Hallucinations

| | | |
|---|---|---|
| Acyclovir | Cycloserine | Metronidazole |
| Albuterol | Cyclosporine | Nalidixic acid |
| Amantadine | Dapsone | Niridazole |
| Aminocaproic acid | Diazepam | Oxymetazoline |
| Amoxicillin | Digitalis | Penicillin |
| Amphetamines | Disopyramide | Pentazocine |
| Anticonvulsants | Disulfiram | Phenylephrine |
| Antidepressants | Ephedrine | Prazosin |
| Antihistamines | Erythromycin | Procainamide |
| Anticholinergics | Ethchlorvynol | Propoxyphene |
| Baclofen | Ethionamide | Propranolol |
| Barbiturates | Gentamicin | Pseudoephedrine |
| Bromocriptine | Indomethacin | Quinacrine |
| Caffeine | Isoniazid | Quinidine |
| Captopril | Ketamine | Salicylates |
| Carbidopa–levodopa | Levodopa | Thiabendazole |
| Chlorambucil | Lidocaine | Thyroid hormone |
| Chloroquine | Maprotiline | Tobramycin |
| Chloramphenicol | Methyldopa | Tocainamide |
| Cimetidine | Methylphenidate | Trazodone |
| Clonazepam | Methysergide | Triazolam |
| Clonidine | Metrizamide | Vincristine |
| Corticosteroids | | |

**Table 9.7**
Hallucinogens

| | |
|---|---|
| LSD (lysergic acid diethylamide) | Harmine |
| Dimethyltryptamine | Mescaline |
| Psilocybin | Tetrahydrocannabinol |
| Psilocin | |

antiparkinsonian agents that up-regulate dopamine metabolism may produce visual hallucinatory states which can be confused with psychiatric diseases. L-dopa and carbidopa/L-dopa combinations may produce psychotic states characterized by vivid, colorful visual hallucinations, which are more prominent at night (Jenkins and Groh, 1970). Thought disorder, agitation, and paranoid features may also be present. Structurally different medications such as buproprion, which may act by inhibiting dopamine uptake, are also capable of producing disorganized psychotic states (Golden *et al.*, 1985). We cannot help but note the pharmacologic irony that dopamine blockers may produce catatonic psychoses, and dopamine agonists may produce noncatatonic psychoses.

The group of drugs which have been called "hallucinogens," "psychotomimetics," "psychodysleptics," and "psychedelics" are listed in Table 9.7. These drugs of abuse have the relatively unusual pharmacologic property of hallucination production in clear consciousness (Baldwin and Hofmann, 1969). Most of these agents are of plant origin and are structurally of some similarity to serotonin. Most abuse of such drugs is done by persons in late adolescence or in their early 20s. At the present time, men are still much more likely than women to abuse them. Psychotic states may supervene after initial use or after more chronic use. The factors that account for this variation are unknown. If any clinical features distinguish hallucinogen-induced psychoses, it might be the plethora of intermixed psychotic features (Ungerleider *et al.*, 1966; Dewhurst and Hatrick, 1972). At least with LSD, multiple colorful visual hallucinations may be intermingled with strange thoughts, auditory hallucinations, and disordered thought process. Cross-modality hallucinations—i.e., "hearing" a color—may be typical of such drugs.

## Checkpoints—Drug and Toxin Hallucinations

### Demographics

Hallucinogen Abuse. Young men.

Antiparkinsonian Drugs. Older patients with history of extrapyramidal disease.

Dopamine-Blocking Drugs. Patients who have been treated for psychoses or for nausea.

## Clinical History

For drug- and toxin-induced psychosis, the aim of the clinical history is straightforward—to ascertain whether the patient may recently have taken drugs from the categories in Table 9.4. Sometimes patients refuse to tell, and sometimes they are unable. In these cases, additional history from families, friends, or observers is essential. Not all patients know the names of drugs or medications they have taken (nor all families), and we have sometimes found it more useful to query after medical conditions treated (e.g., "Did a doctor give you medicine for Parkinson's disease?"). Surprisingly, the time course of clinical onset has not always proved to be of spectacular assistance in diagnosing hallucinations. Most hallucinations, regardless of etiology, have a sudden onset. In our experience, an obsessive approach to the drug history has been the most helpful.

## Psychotropic Drug Interaction

Beware of adding antipsychotic medications to patients with catatonic features. If the catatonia is induced by dopaminergic blockade, such medication will exacerbate it. The risk for neuroleptic malignant syndrome may be heightened.

Monamine oxidase A inhibitors or mixed A and B inhibitors may not be given to patients taking dopamine agonists. The same caveat applies, except for special circumstances, to patients taking antidepressants of tricyclic or heterocyclic structure. When MAO-B inhibitors become available for clinical use, they may be used for such patients in appropriate doses.

## Mental Status Examination

The heterogeneity of the nonparanoid psychoses makes generalization concerning mental status examination patterns difficult. Whether drug-induced catatonic states can be distinguished from psychiatric catatonic states by mental status is dubious. In the hallucinogen- and antiparkinsonian-induced psychoses, the quality of the hallucinations may offer some distinction. Vivid or colorful visual hallucinations appearing in the course of a nonparanoid psychosis should make one suspicious of drug or toxin involvement. Similarly, reports of cross-modality hallucinations, such as seeing sounds or hearing colors, may be clues to LSD or other hallucinogenic abuse.

The key issue during the mental status examination of the hallucinating patient is whether a concurrent encephalopathy exists. If a discernible disruption of arousal, attention, or concentration is present, the clinician must pursue possible toxic and metabolic etiologies tenaciously.

### General Medical Examination

Temperature elevation in catatonia is a worrisome sign, favoring one of the more serious etiologies such as neuroleptic malignant syndrome or CNS infection. Tachycardia and systolic hypertension are seen in drugs that increase catecholamine turnover, such as cocaine, but there is often a generalized sympathetic arousal in all hallucinatory states, including psychiatric.

### Neurologic Examination

Cranial Nerves. Nystagmus—seen in most drug intoxications, including those produced by hallucinogens. Eye movements and optic discs should otherwise be normal, except for limited up-gaze among some parkinsonian patients.

Motor. Increased tone of "waxy" character in catatonic syndromes. Strength should be normal. Coordination may be difficult to test but should not be grossly impaired.

Reflex. Hyperreflexia including clonus and Babinski signs may be seen in some intoxication syndromes. These signs should be symmetric, however.

### Laboratory and Imaging

Imaging. Not of positive diagnostic value in drug-induced syndromes but may "rule out" other etiologies. Do not rush to imaging procedures.

---

*Clinical Rule 9.3:* One thought is worth a thousand CT scans.

---

Laboratory Assays. Hallucinogens—blood or urine assays may be available for THC. Other hallucinogens typically are not tested in toxicology screens. PCP—Blood or urine. Test may remain positive for 7 days after last done.

## METABOLIC DISORDERS ASSOCIATED WITH NONPARANOID PSYCHOSIS

A 45-year-old man worked as a highway supervisor in a rural community. He had no history of psychiatric involvement earlier in life. In the setting of some family system distress surrounding an adolescent child, he developed lethargy and nausea over a period of 3 months. He became forgetful and disorganized in his thinking. On examination, he was pleasant but disoriented and had a major disturbance of thought process. On muscle tone examination he demonstrated waxy flexibility. Serum calcium was 14.6 mg%, and phosphorus was 2.2 mg%.

A 19-year-old man developed symptoms of disordered thinking, depression, and irritability over several weeks. His foreman at his construction job thought that he seemed "slow and disorganized." On interview, he demonstrated prominent difficulty with attention focusing, and persistence. Large-amplitude jerk nystagmus was present on left and right gaze. Muscle tone was diffusely increased. Serum copper was 21 mg/dl (N 70–155) and ceruloplasmin was less than 5 $\mu$g/dl (N 15–50).

A 60-year-old woman developed visual hallucinations, true emotional lability, and disorientation in time and space. On interview, she also had difficulty with attention and persistence. She wept easily but denied depression. Her thought process was tangential but not completely disorganized. Vibratory sensation was completely out at the feet. Her ankle jerks were absent, but knee jerks were brisk. Hemoglobin was 100 g/liter (10 g/dl conventional units). Serum $B_{12}$ was 135 pg/ml ($N > 200$).

As indicated in Table 9.4, we have selected a limited number of metabolic disorders to review in this chapter; hypercalcemic states, Wilson's disease, hepatic encephalopathy, and certain deficiency states. Such a list is obviously too short, since if extreme, any metabolic disturbance is capable of disrupting thought process, perception, and muscle tone. It is our judgment and experience, however, that these four etiologies come under consideration in psychiatric patients relatively more frequently than others. Psychiatric clinicians need to have at least an initial diagnostic familiarity with them.

The first vignette above describes a patient who ultimately proved to have a pancreatic carcinoma with circulating parathyroidlike peptides and resultant hyperparathyroidism, hypercalcemia, and hypophosphatemia. Such a clinical picture has been reported in hyperparathyroidism secondary to parathyroid adenoma (Hockaday *et al.*, 1966), and we suspect that it can be produced by hypercalcemia of any etiology. Hypercalcemia may be present upon screening laboratory testing from a variety of etiologies. It is important for clinicians to remember that calcium is heavily bound to serum albumin, so that artifactual elevations or depressions of serum calcium may appear when albumin levels are high or low. A good rule with regard to patients with low serum albumin is to subtract 1 mg/dl from the serum calcium concentration for every 1.0 g/dl the serum albumin is lower than 4.0 g/dl.

Wilson's disease is an autosomally recessively inherited disease of copper metabolism. It is a rare disease, with lifetime prevalence rates ranging from 5 to 30 per million, most of which are probably unrecognized. Wilson's disease is important to psychiatrists because it affects young people, is treatable, and may present with behavioral manifestations (Dening, 1985; Chung *et al.*, 1986; Cartwright, 1978; Goldstein *et al.*, 1968). Dening reviewed the behavioral disturbances reported in the medical literature as of 1985 and remarked on the great variety of syndromes and symptoms that may be seen, ranging from affective disorders through psychotic states to dementia. We have included Wilson's disease in this chapter because of the multiform psychiatric disturbances associated with it, not because there is one typical, nonparanoid psychotic profile that can provide clinicians with a fake sense of security.

Hepatic encephalopathy is another common cause of disturbed thought and perception (Summerskill *et al.*, 1956; Reed, *et al.*, 1967). A variety of pathophysiologic states may produce hepatic failure, including viral infections, alcohol abuse, malignancies, and some medications. When this process is early, however, the patients may present with predominantly mental status syndromes. These patients are encephalopathic, and on mental status examination, they demonstrate special difficulties with tasks involving attention and concentration. Characteristic physical findings including asterixis may be present, as well as stigmata of the underlying liver disease. Venous or arterial ammonia is usually elevated, as is CSF glutamine (Fraser and Arieff, 1985).

We are including the mental status syndromes associated with deficiencies of $B_{12}$ and possibly folate in this chapter, although no single profile of mental disturbance can be considered typical. A range of disorganized psychotic states have been reported in people with these syndromes, as well as affective and paranoid disturbances (Strachun and Henderson, 1965; Shulman, 1972; Roos, 1978; Evans *et al.*, 1983). Again, a variety of mental status abnormalities have been described. Depressive syndromes have been reported, as well as bizarre behavior, disordered thought processes, and true emotional lability. We have seen such patients and have *not* been impressed with obvious delirious features. Most of these patients *do*, however, have neurologic findings such as peripheral neuropathy. The peripheral blood parameters need not demonstrate anemia. Macrocytosis and the presence of hypersegmented polymorphonuclear neutrophils have been more reliable in our experience. Serum $B_{12}$ levels and Schilling's tests are required for diagnosis. It has been more difficult to adduce definite evidence of an etiologic link between folate deficiency and behavioral disturbance (Reynolds, 1976). Low serum folate in the presence of normal serum $B_{12}$ may occur in patients suffering from malabsorption syndromes and patients taking phenytoin or phenobarbital. Since folate replacement in a $B_{12}$-deficient patient may correct the macrocytosis without affecting the neuropathology, it is wise to be meticulous in evaluating $B_{12}$ metabolism before prescribing folate replacement.

Finally, within this category of metabolic disease and nonparanoid psychosis, we have included pellagra, a deficiency syndrome that we hope will prove of only historical interest. In the days before routine supplementation of manufactured bread with nicotinic acid, some people who had subsisted on diets predominantly of starchy vegetables through the winter became psychotic in the spring (Spies *et al.*, 1938; Slater, 1942). In a time when unusual diets may be practiced by certain subcultures of society, psychiatric clinicians should know some of their own history in this regard. The psychoses of nicotinic acid deficiency tended to be of the disorganized type clinically, were associated with unusual diets as noted above, and typically occurred in the presence of sustained diarrhea, stomatitis, and dermatitis over sun-exposed areas. There is no laboratory test for niacin deficiency. These syndromes still occur, particularly among patients who are alcoholic, on fad diets, or taking isoniazid (Spivak and Jackson, 1977).

## Demographics

Wilson's disease typically onsets in childhood or early adult life. The sexes are affected equally.

Hyperparathyroidism is most common in women over the age of 60. Men are affected at lesser rates, and young adults may be affected.

The demographics of the hepatic syndrome depend on a variety of underlying liver diseases, although alcoholism probably leads the list.

Patients who have undergone partial or total gastrectomies are at greater risk for developing $B_{12}$ deficiency syndromes, since the intrinsic transport factor is located in the gastric antrum. Patients with blind loop GI anatomy (such as after Bilroth II operations) are also at risk. Alcoholics and epileptics on phenytoin and phenobarbital are at risk for folate deficiency.

## Clinical History

When one considers these metabolic syndromes and nonparanoid psychoses, there are often obvious clues in the clinical history (i.e., previously diagnosed malignancy in some hypercalcemic states; known alcoholism with cirrhosis). When such features are not present, one attempts to elicit clues from the clinical history that an underlying metabolic problem may be present. Has there been nausea or vomiting? Abdominal pain? Lethargy? Abnormal movements witnessed by observers? A strange diet that could potentiate B-complex or folate deficiency? Weight loss? Family history of neurologic or psychiatric disease with onset in young adulthood? (Families do not usually announce that they have Wilson's disease.) Many of these questions are part of any thorough medical history, as opposed to specific probes for specific diseases. As we have emphasized before, much caution is warranted with the nonparanoid psychoses, in view of the wide array of medical conditions that may produce them.

## Psychotropic Drug Interactions

None specific.

## Mental Status Examination

We suspect that many of the catatonic as well as the more disorganized psychotic states associated with these medical and neurological diseases are actually mild encephalopathic states. Careful examination of orientation, arousal, and concentration is warranted. Unfortunately, we have no clinical research to indicate that the psychiatric diseases may not also impair these mental status functions, and our clinical impression is that they can. In nonparanoid psychoses, the mental status examination alone is not a reliable diagnostic guide. Fortunately, the physical examination is always positive.

*Clinical Rule 9.4:* In a nonparanoid psychosis, if you must choose between the interview and the examination, pick the examination.

## General Medical Examination

HEENT. Kayser-Fleischer rings are present in more than 90% of people with Wilson's disease. These appear as brown, green, or yellow pigmentation as a ring at the periphery of the cornea. They may sometimes be seen by cross-illuminating the cornea in a darkened room, but slit-lamp examination by an ophthalmologist may be needed.

Skin. Note punctate spider angiomata in cirrhosis, or icteric cast. In nicotinic acid deficiency syndromes, erythematous rash may be evident in sun-exposed areas.

GI. Check for hepatomegaly, nodularity, tenderness. Ileus may be present in hypercalcemic states. Remember that Wilson's disease may cause cirrhosis.

## Neurologic Examination

Cranial Nerves. Kayser-Fleischer rings are described in the previous section. Dysarthria and dysphagia may be prominent early in Wilson's disease. In a recent series of 31 Wilson's patients, dysarthria was present in 90% (Starosta-Rubinstein *et al.*, 1987). Patients with early hepatic encephalopathy almost always demonstrate abnormalities of extraocular muscle movements; nystagmus, overshoot dysmetria as the eyes swing to a target, saccadic pursuits as a target is tracked.

Motor Bulk. One should develop a sense for atrophy such as may be seen in deficiency states.

*Tone.* May be increased in Wilson's disease, typically with "lead pipe" quality.

*Power.* Proximal muscle weakness may be seen in hypercalcemia.

*Coordination.* Wilson's patients may be ataxic and dysmetric on finger-to-nose, heel-to-shin, and gait testing. Hepatic encephalopathy patients typically demonstrate such abnormalities.

*Abnormal movements.* Note tremor especially, which is common in Wilson's disease. It may be parkinsonian, or it may be large-amplitude, "wing beating" in pattern. Asterixis is common in hepatic encephalopathy. One should recall that electrophysiologically, asterixis is due to sudden, brief lapses in postural muscle tone, so that the extended hand or fingers seem to suddenly "drop" until they are "caught" and returned to position. Sometimes the finding can be felt by gently holding the patient's hand and fingers in extension.

Reflex. Hyperreflexia and Babinski signs may be seen in Wilson's disease.

## Laboratory and Imaging

Hyperparathyroidism. Elevation of serum calcium is most reliable finding. Normal ranges for calcium:

| | | |
|---|---|---|
| Male | 8.8–10.3 mg/dl | 2.20–2.58 mmole/liter |
| Female (< 50 yrs) | 8.8–10.0 mg/dl | 2.20–2.50 mmole/liter |
| Female (> 50 yrs) | 8.8–10.2 mg/dl | 2.20–2.56 mmole/liter |

Repeated measurements should be made to confirm a pattern of elevated levels. Low serum phosphate is often present and is supportive of the diagnosis. Urinary calcium excretion may actually be decreased in hyperparathyroidism. A radioimmunoassay for parathyroid hormone may be sent next. This is often, but not always, elevated.

Hypercalcemia may also appear in the course of malignancies (particularly lung), vitamin D intoxication, long-term ingestion of milk and antacids, thyrotoxicoses, adrenal insufficiency, and sarcoidosis.

Hepatic Syndromes. Hyperammonemia is usually present in patients with hepatic encephalopathy:

| | | |
|---|---|---|
| $NH_3$ | 10–80 $\mu$g/dl | (5–50 $\mu$mole/liter) |
| $NH_4$ | 10–85 $\mu$g/dl | (5–50 $\mu$mole/liter) |
| Nitrogen | 10–65 $\mu$g/dl | (5–50 $\mu$mole/liter) |

The ammonia is not always elevated, however, and may not itself be the neurotoxin. Arterial ammonia is probably the most reliable, although venous ammonia drawn without the use of a tourniquet is also satisfactory.

### $B_{12}$ Deficiency

*Serum $B_{12}$ level.* The lowest tolerated serum $B_{12}$ level determined by *L. leichmannii* assay has been fixed at 200 pg/ml by the WHO.

*Schilling test.* A tracer dose of $B_{12}$ labeled with $^{58}CO$ is given orally. Two hours later, 1 mg of nonradioactive $B_{12}$ is given IM, with the result that much of the absorbed radioactive $B_{12}$ is excreted in urine. In patients unable to absorb $B_{12}$ orally, a low percentage of labeled $B_{12}$ is excreted. The test may be repeated with intrinsic factor. A 24-hr urine must be collected as part of this test, so patients must be cooperative. In addition, serum $B_{12}$ determinations are distorted by the injection of $B_{12}$ and so should be determined prior to performance of the Schilling test.

Wilson's Disease. Serum ceruloplasmin is decreased ($<$ 20 mg/100 ml), serum copper is decreased, urinary copper is elevated, and free amino acids are present in urine. Liver enzymes (alkaline phosphatase, ALT, AST, GGTP) are often elevated, too, but are not specific. Head MR scans may show increased signal intensity in basal ganglia and in other brain areas.

## TUMOR, TRAUMA, AND NONPARANOID PSYCHOSIS

Clinicians do not typically consider an important association between either CNS tumor or trauma and psychosis. We expect tumors to produce focal neurologic findings and trauma to produce the "posttraumatic" syndromes of altered consciousness and cognition, along with focal neurologic damage when more severe. Both groups should demonstrate major cognitive disturbances. Both of these principles tend to hold true. But for those clinicians who forget the following clinical rules, we will provide a brief review of literature in this area.

---

*Clinical Rule 9.5:* Dementia cannot be found until the mental status examination is conducted.

*Clinical Rule 9.6:* Focal neurologic findings are certain to be missed if the patient is not examined.

---

Psychotic mental syndromes have been reported following both penetrating and nonpenetrating brain injury (Achte *et al.*, 1969; Hillbom and Kaila,

1951; Filley and Jarvis, 1987). Some of these syndromes are similar to the disorganized psychoses, although these are often obvious associated cognitive impairments and focal neurologic findings. Hillbom's group reported that schizophreniform symptomatology was more likely to be associated with brain injury that affected the temporal lobes. We have commonly seen closed-head injury patients pass through a period of amnestic disorganized psychosis after consciousness has returned. These patients are rarely confused with psychiatric syndromes diagnostically, since the history of trauma is obvious. Catatonia does not usually occur in these patients. There are also anecdotal reports of schizophreniform psychotic states appearing after more minor closed-head injuries. We have not encountered such a syndrome in our clinical experience, and we wonder if such events do not report coincidental phenomena.

In large autopsy series, there is evidence that psychiatric patients demonstrate a greater number of unsuspected brain tumors than do medical controls (Raskin, 1956; Patton and Sheppard, 1956). The elevation in tumor rates is not large, on the order of 3.7% versus 2.3% in nonpsychiatric patients. In addition, most of these data come from the preneuroimaging era, before the advent of CT and MR scanning. Meningiomas tend to be the tumor most commonly identified.

Lishman (1978) has pointed out that hallucinatory symptoms tend to be related to hemispheric brain tumors, with the quality of the hallucination depending somewhat on the location of the tumor. Occipital lobe tumors may produce unformed visual hallucinations, temporal lobe tumors, more complex visual and auditory hallucinations, and parietal lobe tumors, tactile or kinesthetic sensory alterations. In our experience, frontal lobe tumors, especially the higher-grade gliomas, tend to produce blunting or disinhibition of the personality, which is not usually mistaken for psychosis. When more advanced, these frontal lobe tumor patients may demonstrate catatonic features.

## Demographics

**Head Trauma.** Most likely to occur among young men, although no one is immune. Events are usually self-evident.

**Tumor.** Meningiomas account for approximately half of primary brain tumors associated with behavioral change. They are slow-growing, circumscribed tumors that occur two or three times more commonly in women than in men. The fifth and sixth decades are the most likely years of onset.

## Clinical History

A history of head trauma is usually self-evident. In tumor patients, however, the clues and cues to be listened for may be more subtle. Has there been a concomitant change in personality? Common patterns of behavioral change we have observed include a progressive disinhibition of social mores and behavior, or a progressive apathy and social withdrawal not associated with a true affective disturbance. Such changes may take the form of progressive carelessness in personal appearance, loss of capacity to feel shame or guilt, loss of impulse control which had previously been present, and similar phenomena. Headache is a helpful clue when spontaneously offered by the patient (as opposed to a response to direct question). Memory disturbance has been reported as a complaint in tumor patients, as have language disturbance and seizure.

## Psychotropic Drug Interaction

None specific.

## Mental Status Examination

Both trauma and tumor produce cognitive disturbance, the pattern depending somewhat on severity of trauma or location of tumor. Serial performance tasks of attention and concentration may be quite sensitive in both conditions. Verbal and visual memory may also be disturbed in either syndrome. Tumors can produce a variety of other cognitive impairments, depending on location.

## General Medical Examination

Palpate and inspect scalp for signs of trauma. Are these areas of bleeding ecchymosis, tenderness? Tenderness to tapping or percussion sometimes occurs over a brain tumor or over a subdural hematoma. Again, the sign is more valuable if spontaneously reported by the patient.

## Neurological Examination

Cranial Nerves. Papilledema or loss of spontaneous venous pulsations should be checked. The venous pulses are most easily seen at proximal bends in the vessels. In early papilledema the vessels may be obscured as they emerge from the disc. Extraocular muscle palsies and field defects should also be checked.

Sensory. Not usually of great sensitivity or specificity.

### Motor

*Tone*. Subtle asymmetry of tone may be a warning sign concerning hemispheric lesions.

*Power.* Before overt weakness is apparent, there may be external rotation of a leg during gait testing, or a positive pronator drift. Fine finger movements may be slowed or clumsy early on the side opposite a hemispheric tumor.

*Reflex.* Again, asymmetry is important to identify.

### Laboratory and Imaging

Head CT scan remains the imaging gold standard for both traumatic syndromes and tumor, although MR technology is becoming widely available and provides partly complementary information. Contrast injection for an enhanced scan is not routinely necessary. In trauma syndromes one is usually seeking evidence of swelling or hemorrhage, neither of which requires enhancement. More than 90% of tumors are evident on unenhanced scans, and we prefer to reserve enhancement for cases in which the likelihood of such a lesion is high. The occasional allergies or renal reactions to contrast enhancement confer a sense of humility on the ordering physician if the test was not truly necessary.

## EPILEPSY AND NONPARANOID PSYCHOSIS

A 65-year-old woman had undergone five previous psychiatric admissions for treatment of unipolar depression earlier in her life. During dinner with her daughter, she suddenly stopped speaking, undressed herself, and lay on the floor. She refused to explain this behavior. Later in the meal, she loudly and abruptly exclaimed, "I'm dying . . . I'm bleeding from the nose!" When brought to the emergency room she was generally coherent, with periods of mutism. Occasional twitching movements of the left side of the face were observed. An EEG showed continuous bilateral delta activity over both hemispheres with scattered runs of spike wave and multiple spike discharges.

Nonconvulsive status epilepticus is a syndrome that typically occurs in middle to late life and which appears clinically like a disorganized behavioral state (Van Rossum *et al.*, 1985; Lee, 1985; Guberman *et al.*, 1986). As reflected in the vignette above, the behavior typically includes features of thought process disorganization, mutism, stereotypical behaviors, or eccentric behaviors. There is often a clinical history of previous epilepsy, although this need not always be present, especially in the more elderly, where small vascular lesions probably generate the epileptic foci. Most of the patients described in the reports cited had abnormalities on neurologic examination—focal signs of underlying structural brain disease, or at least fleeting clinical signs of continuing seizure discharge. Similarly, most of these patients demonstrated cognitive abnormalities, such as depressed arousal, amnestic syndromes, and disorientation.

Individual seizures, as opposed to partial status epilepticus, may produce isolated psychotic symptoms (Lowall, 1976). The most common such ictal symptoms include intermittent confusion or thought blocking, mutism, and hallucinations, with olfactory hallucinations the most common. As with the episodes of nonconvulsive status, most of these patients have either epileptic histories or subtle examination evidence for seizure discharge.

## Demographics

Partial complex epilepsy is the type of epilepsy most often associated with psychoticlike clinical features. There are two age peaks of clinical onset for this type of epilepsy: early adult life from late adolescence to the early 20s, and late adult life, such as the seventh decade. The pathophysiology probably differs between the two age peaks, with residual congenital lesions accounting for the earlier cases, and small vascular lesions underlying the later one. Partial complex seizures can always be considered to occur secondary to some underlying neurologic lesion, such as mesial temporal sclerosis, stroke, or tumor.

## Clinical History

Some people (or their families) do not like to admit to "seizures," "fits," or "convulsions." "Spell" or "faint" may be more acceptable terms, and sometimes one must use indirection, asking about memory lapses, nocturnal incontinence, and lip-smacking. Again, it is worth remembering that the great majority of patients with ictal psychotic symptoms have had previous epileptic events, whether diagnosed or not.

## Psychotropic Drug Interactions

See discussion under Epilepsy in Chapter 8. All antipsychotic drugs lower seizure threshold, although the effect size is drug- and dose-dependent. Among antidepressants the effect on seizure threshold is minimal, except for maprotiline.

## Mental Status Examination

**Arousal.** Typically impaired or interrupted during nonconvulsive status or during postictal period. One should especially observe sudden lapses of attention, after which the patient is momentarily confused.

**Orientation.** Also likely to be transiently disturbed.

### General Medical Examination

Nonspecific.

### Neurological Examination

Observe perioral and periocular musculature carefully. A relatively broad area of cerebral cortex controls facial and periorbital musculature, and even partial seizures will typically "spill over" into these areas. The same principle applies to hands and fingers. When clinical suspicion rises, one should observe these areas carefully for a period of minutes. The ictal movements may be transient.

### Laboratory and Imaging

EEG is the definitive test. Most patients with nonconvulsive status epilepticus have demonstrated continuous runs of spike-wave discharge.

## CNS INFECTION AND NONPARANOID PSYCHOSIS

Viral encephalitis almost always compromises mental status function and may occasionally present as a disorganized psychosis (Shearer, 1964). Herpes simplex is the most common nonseasonal cause of encephalitis and typically includes features of disorientation, fluctuating arousal, and (interestingly) catatonia (Raskin, 1974). The virus causes a focal encephalitis, involving temporal and basal frontal lobes, which probably accounts for the limbic clinical features that sometimes occur. Usually the behavioral symptomatology occurs in the context of a fulminant infectious illness, and true diagnostic uncertainty with regard to psychiatric illness is either rare or transient.

Himmelhoch *et al.* (1970) and Misra and Hay (1971) have described a more subacute viral encephalitis, presenting with features of disorganized psychosis and delirium. Most of these patients had abnormal spinal fluid examinations, but specific infectious agents were not identified. We have not encountered such a syndrome.

Today, the human immune deficiency virus is the infectious agent most often considered in the diagnostic evaluation of behavioral change. Certain high-risk groups, including male homosexuals, IV drug abusers, and patients who have received transfusions, are more likely to develop the syndrome, but no group is "immune." In most of these cases, the antibody to the virus can be detected in serum, and either CSF or neuroimaging tests are abnormal. The virus can also be identified or cultured from CSF at specialized centers.

### Demographics

High-risk groups for HIV infection: (1) male homosexuals; (2) IV drug abusers; (3) persons who have received transfusions; (4) hemophiliacs; and (5) children of high-risk parents.

For non-HIV encephalitis, there may be a seasonal epidemic pattern. Predisposing factors for herpes encephalitis are not known.

### General Medical Examination

It is embarrassing when an encephalitic patient is evaluated and the temperature is not taken. These patients (except the HIV patients) are usually febrile. Vital signs, taken routinely, remain the best screening measure for infected patients.

### Laboratory and Imaging

When encephalitis becomes a clinical consideration, lumbar puncture, EEG, and CT/MR become the tests of choice. Viruses cannot be cultured quickly, from CSF, unlike bacteria, but pleocytosis and elevated protein can be identified. Many patients with HIV syndromes involving CNS also have elevated IgG in CSF and oligoclonal banding of IgG on protein electrophoresis.

## ENDOCRINE DISORDERS AND NONPARANOID PSYCHOSIS

We have discussed clinical reports of catatonia associated with hyperparathyroidism under the "Delirium" section. Those syndromes are probably mediated by the hypercalcemia. There are other reports of simple and catatonic schizophreniform syndromes associated with thyrotoxicoses (Bursten, 1961). These are not typical features for thyrotoxicosis, which is more likely to appear with affective signs or symptoms and is discussed more fully in those chapters.

## STROKE AND NONPARANOID PSYCHOSIS

Large-vessel stroke is almost never confused with psychiatric syndromes. The only exception worth considering is dominant hemisphere middle cerebral artery strokes, which affect Wernicke's area but spare obvious motor functions. Acute onset of such a receptive aphasia may occasionally appear as a disorganized psychosis. Posterior right-hemisphere stroke may also occasionally present as an agitated psychosis (Pakalnis *et al.*, 1987). For all of these vascular syndromes, recognizing risk factors in the clinical situations (hypertension; other evidence for atherosclerosis) and performing a cognitive assessment should be sufficient to avoid diagnostic errors.

## ARTERITIS

A last comment is made in this chapter concerning the perils of missing giant cell (temporal) arteritis in the elderly. This eminently treatable inflammatory condition afflicts the elderly (almost all cases are among patients in the seventh decade or later) and is part of a systemic illness picture. Common signs and symptoms include fever, myalgias, weight loss, night sweats, liver dysfunction, and headache. Hallucinatory symptoms occasionally appear (Hart, 1967). The erythrocyte sedimentation rate is almost always elevated, and this test is probably worth checking on all elderly patients with new behavioral syndromes.

## REFERENCES


Abrams, R., and Taylor, M. A. Catatonia; a prospective clinical study. *Arch. Gen. Psychiatry*, 1976, **33,** 579–581.

Achte, K. A., Hillbom, E., and Aalberg, V. Psychoses following war brain injuries. *Acta Psychiatr. Scand.*, 1969, **45,** 1–18.

Andreasen, N. C., Smith, M. R., Jacoby, C. G., Dennert, J. W., and Olsen, S. A. Ventricular enlargement in schizophrenia: Definition and prevalence. *Am. J. Psychiatry*, 1982a, **139,** 292–296.

Andreasen, N. C., Olsen, S. A., Dennert, J. W., and Smith, M. R. Ventricular enlargement in schizophrenia: Relationship to positive and negative symptoms. *Am. J. Psychiatry*, 1982b, **139,** 297–302.

Baldwin, M., and Hofmann, A. Hallucinations. In Vinken, P. J., and Bruyn, G. W. (eds.): *Handbook of Clinical Neurology*. Amsterdam: North-Holland, 1969, pp. 327–339.

Bursten, B. Psychoses associated with thyrotoxicosis. *Arch. Gen. Psychiatry*, 1961, **4,** 267–273.

Cartwright, G. E. Diagnosis of treatable Wilson's disease. *N. Engl. J. Med.*, 1978, **298,** 1347–1350.

Chung, Y. S., Ravi, S. D., and Borge, G. F. Psychosis in Wilson's disease. *Psychosomatics*, 1986, **27,** 65–66.

Dening, T. R. Psychiatric aspects of Wilson's disease. *Br. J. Psychiatry*, 1985, **147,** 677–682.

Dewhurst, K., and Hatrick, J. A. Differential diagnosis and treatment of lysergic acid diethylamide induced psychosis. *Practitioner*, 1972, **209,** 327–332.

*Diagnostic and Statistical Manual of Mental Disorders*, 3d ed., revised. Washington, D.C.: American Psychiatric Association, 1987.

Ebaugh, F. G., Barnacle, C. H., and Ewalt, J. P. Delirious episodes associated with artificial fever. *Am. J. Psychiatry*, 1936, **93,** 191–217.

Engel, G. L., and Romano, J. Delirium, a syndrome of cerebral insufficiency. *J. Chron. Dis.*, 1959, **9,** 260–277.

Evans, D. L., Edelsohn, G. A., and Golden, R. N. Organic psychosis without anemia or spinal cord symptoms in patients with vitamin $B_{12}$ deficiency. *Am. J. Psychiatry*, 1983, **140,** 218–221.

Filley, C. M., and Jarvis, P. E. Delayed reduplicative paramnesia. *Neurology (NY)*, 1987, **37,** 701–703.

Fraser, C. L., and Arieff, A. I. Hepatic encephalopathy. *N. Engl. J. Med.*, 1985, **313,** 865–873.

Gelenberg, A. J. The catatonic syndrome. *Lancet*, 1976, **1,** 1339–1341.

Geller, T. J., and Bellur, S. N. Peduncular hallucinosis: Magnetic resonance imaging confirmation of mesencephalic infarction during life. *Ann. Neurol.*, 1987, **21,** 602–604.

Golden, C. J., Moses, J. A. Jr., Zelazowski, R., Graber, B., Zatz, L. M., Horvath, T. B., and Berger, P. A. Cerebral ventricular size and neuropsychological impairment in young chronic schizophrenics. *Arch. Gen. Psychiatry*, 1980, **37,** 619–623.

Golden, R. N., James, S. P., Sherer, M. A., Rudorfer, M. V., Sack, D. A., and Potter, W. Z. Psychoses associated with buproprion treatment. *Am. J. Psychiatry*, 1985, **142,** 1459–1462.

Goldstein, N. P., Ewert, G. C., Randall, R. V., and Gross, J. B. Psychiatric aspects of Wilson's disease (hepatolenticular degeneration): Results of psychometric tests during long term therapy. *Am. J. Psychiatry*, 1968, **124,** 1555–1561.

Guberman, A., Cantu-Reyna, G., Stuss, D., and Broughton, R. Nonconvulsive generalized status epilepticus: Clinical features, neuropsychological testing, and long-term follow-up. *Neurology (NY)*, 1986, **36,** 1284–1291.

Hanes, E. L. Acute delerium in psychiatric practice, with special reference to so-called acute delirious mania (collapse delirium). *J. Nerv. Ment. Dis.*, 1912, **39,** 236–250.

Hart, C. T. Formed visual hallucinations: A symptom of cranial arteritis. *Br. Med. J.*, 1967, **3,** 643–644.

Herman, M., Harpham, D., and Rosenblum, M. Nonschizophrenic catatonic states. *N. Y. State J. Med.*, 1942, **42,** 624–627.

Hillbom, E., and Kaila, M. Schizophrenia-like psychoses after brain trauma. *Acta Psychiatr. Neurol.*, 1951, (Suppl. 60), 36–47.

Himmelhoch, J., Pincus, J., Tucker, G., and Peter, D. Subacute encephalitis: Behavioral and neurologic aspects. *Br. J. Psychiatry*, 1970, **116,** 531–538.

Hockaday, T. D. R., Keynes, W. M., and McKenzie, J. K. Catatonic stupor in an elderly woman with hyperparathyroidism. *Br. Med. J.*, 1966, **1,** 85–87.

Jenkins, R. B., and Groh, R. H. Mental symptoms in parkinsonian patients treated with L-dopa. *Lancet*, 1970, **2,** 177–180.

Kahlbaum, K. L. *Catatonia* (1874). Translated by George Mora. Baltimore: Johns Hopkins University Press, 1973.

Lee, I. Nonconvulsive status epilepticus. *Arch. Neurol.*, 1985, **42,** 778–781.

Lipowski, Z. J. Delirium, clouding of consciousness and confusion. *J. Nerv. Ment. Dis.*, 1967, **145,** 227–255.

Lipowski, Z. J. Delirium (acute confusional states). *JAMA*, 1987, **258,** 1789–1792.

Lishman, W. A. *Organic Psychiatry: The Psychological Consequences of Cerebral Disorder*. Oxford, U.K.: Blackwell Scientific, 1978.

Lowall, J. Psychiatric presentations of seizures. *Am. J. Psychiatry*, 1976, **133,** 321–323.

Luchins, D. J., Weinberger, D. R., and Wyatt, R. J. Schizophrenia and cerebral asymmetry detected by computed tomography. *Am. J. Psychiatry*, 1982, **139,** 753–757.

Mann, S. C., Caroff, S. N., Bleier, H. R., Welz, W. K. R., Kling, M. A., and Hayashida, M. Lethal catatonia. *Am. J. Psychiatry*, 1986, **143,** 1374–1381.

McGucken, R. B., and Caldwell, J. Teenage procyclidine abuse. *Lancet*, 1985, **1,** 1514 (letter).

Medical Letter. Drugs that cause psychiatric symptoms. *Med. Lett. Drugs Ther.*, 1986, **28,** 81–86.

Medina, J. L., Chokroverty, S., and Rubino, F. A. Syndrome of agitated delirium and visual impairment: A manifestation of medial temporo-occipital infarction. *J. Neurol. Neurosurg. Psychiatry*, 1977, **40,** 861–864.

*Mental Disorders: Glossary and Guide to Their Classification in Accordance with the Ninth Revision of the International Classification of Diseases.* Geneva: World Health Organization, 1978.

Mesulam, M., Waxman, S. G., Geschwind, N., and Sabin, T. D. Acute confusional states with right middle cerebral artery infarctions. *J. Neurol. Neurosurg. Psychiatry*, 1976, **39,** 84–89.

Misra, P. C., and Hay, G. G. Encephalitis presenting as acute schizophrenia. *Br. Med. J.*, 1971, **1,** 532–533.

Nasrallah, H. A., Jacoby, C. G., McCalley-Whitters, M., and Kuperman, S. Cerebral ventricular enlargement in subtypes of chronic schizophrenia. *Arch. Gen. Psychiatry*, 1982, **39,** 774–777.

Newmann, M. A. Periventricular diffuse pinealoma. Report of a case with clinical features of catatonic schizophrenia. *J. Nerv. Ment. Dis.*, 1955, **121,** 193–204.

Nicholi, A. M. The nontherapeutic use of psychoactive drugs. *N. Engl. J. Med.*, 1983, **308,** 925–933.

Pakalnis, A., Drake, M. E., and Kellum, T. B. Right parieto-occipital lacunar infarction with agitation, hallucinations, and delusions. *Psychosomatics*, 1987, **28,** 95–96.

Patton, R. B., and Sheppard, J. A. Intracranial tumors found at autopsy in mental patients. *Am. J. Psychiatry*, 1956, **113,** 319–324.

Penn, H., Racy J., Lapham, L., Mandel, M., and Sandt, J. Catatonic behavior, viral encephalopathy, and death. *Arch. Gen. Psychiatry*, 1972, **27,** 758–761.

Quitkin, F., Rifkin, A., and Klein, D. F. Neurologic soft signs in schizophrenia and character disorders. *Arch. Gen. Psychiatry*, 1976, **33,** 845–853.

Raskin, D. E., and Frank, S. W. Herpes encephalitis with catatonic stupor. *Arch. Gen. Psychiatry*, 1974, **31,** 544–546.

Raskin, N. Intracranial neoplasms in psychotic patients. *Am. J. Psychiatry*, 1956, **112,** 481–484.

Reed, A. E., Sherlock, S., Laidlaw, J., and Walker, J. G. The neuropsychiatric syndromes associated with chronic liver disease and an extensive portal–systemic collateral circulation. *Q. J. Med.*, 1967, **36,** 135–150.

Reynolds, E. H. Neurological aspects of folate and vitamin $B_{12}$ metabolism. *Clin. Haematol.*, 1976, **5,** 661–696.

Rochford, J. M., Detre, T., Tucker, G. J., and Harrow, M. Neuropsychological impairments in functional psychiatric diseases. *Arch. Gen. Psychiatry*, 1970, **22,** 114–119.

Rogers, D. The motor disorders of severe psychiatric illness: A conflict of paradigms. *Br. J. Psychiatry*, 1985, **147,** 221–232.

Roos, D. Neurological complications in patients with impaired vitamin $B_{12}$ absorption following partial gastrectomy. *Acta Neurol. Scand.*, 1978, **59** (Suppl. 69), 1–77.

Schwab, J. J., and Barrow, M. V. A reaction to organic fluorides simulating classical catatonia. *Am. J. Psychiatry*, 1964, **120,** 1196–1197.

Shader, R. I. *Psychiatric Complications of Medical Drugs.* New York: Raven Press, 1972.

Shearer, M. L., and Finch, S. M. Periodic organic psychosis associated with recurrent herpes simplex. *N. Engl. J. Med.*, 1964, **271,** 494–497.

Shulman, R. The recent status of vitamin $B_{12}$ and folic acid deficiency in psychiatric illness. *Can. Psychiatr. Assoc. J.*, 1972, **17,** 205–216.

Slater, E. Psychosis associated with vitamin B deficiency. *Br. Med. J.*, 1942, **1,** 257–258.

Spies, T. D., Aring, C. D., Gelperin, J., and Bean, W. B. The mental symptoms of pellagra: Their relief with nicotinic acid. *Am. J. Med. Sci.*, 1938, **196,** 461–475.

Spivak, J. L., and Jackson, D. L. Pellagra: An analysis of 18 patients and a review of the literature. *Johns Hopkins Med. J.*, 1977, **140,** 295–309.

Starosta-Rubinstein, S., Young, A. B., Kluin, K., Hill, G., Aisen, A. M., Gabrielsen, T., and Brewer, G. J. Clinical assessment of 31 patients with Wilson's disease: Correlations with structural changes on magnetic resonance imaging. *Arch. Neurol.*, 1987, **44,** 365–370.

Stoudemire, A. The differential diagnosis of catatonic states. *Psychosomatics*, 1982, **23,** 245–252.

Strachun, R. W., and Henderson, J. G. Psychiatric syndromes due to avitaminosis $B_{12}$ with normal blood and marrow. *Q. J. Med.*, 1965, **34,** 303–317.

Summerskill, W. H. J., Davidson, E. A., Sherlock, S., and Steiner, R. E. The neuropsychiatric syndrome associated with hepatic cirrhosis and an extensive portal collateral circulation. *Q. J. Med.*, 1956, **25,** 245–266.

Sunderland, T., Tariot, P. N., Cohen, R. M., Weingartner, H., Mueller, E. A., and Murphy, D. L. Anticholinergic sensitivity in patients with dementia of the Alzheimer type and age-matched controls. *Arch. Gen. Psychiatry*, 1987, **44,** 418–426.

Tippin, J., and Dunner, F. J. Biparietal infarctions in a patient with catatonia. *Am. J. Psychiatry*, 1981, **138,** 1386–1387.

Tsai, L. Y., Nasrallah, H. A., and Jacoby, C. G. Hemispheric asymmetries on computed tomographic scans in schizophrenia and mania. *Arch. Gen. Psychiatry*, 1983, **40,** 1286–1289.

Ungerleider, J. T., Fisher, D. D., and Fuller, M. The dangers of LSD. *JAMA*, 1966, **197,** 389–392.

Van Rossum, J., Groeneveld-Ockhuysen, A. A. W., and Arts, R. J. H. M. Psychomotor status. *Arch. Neurol.*, 1985, **42,** 989–993.

Weinberger, D. R. Implications of normal brain development for the pathogenesis of schizophrenia. *Arch. Gen. Psychiatry*, 1987, **44,** 660–669.

Weinberger, D. R., Bigelow, L. B., and Kleinman, J. E. Cerebral ventricular enlargement in chronic schizophrenia: An association with poor response to treatment. *Arch. Gen. Psychiatry*, 1980, **37,** 11–13.

Weinreb, H. J. Saccadic intrusions in schizophrenia: Identity with square-wave jerks? *Arch. Gen. Psychiatry*, 1983, **40,** 1343 (letter).

Wolff, H. G., and Curran, D. Nature of delirium and allied states. *Arch. Neurol. Psychiatry*, 1935, **33,** 1175–1215.

Woods, S. W. Catatonia in patients with subdural hematomas. *Am. J. Psychiatry*, 1980, **137,** 983–984.

# Index

GPSR Compliance

*The European Union's (EU) General Product Safety Regulation (GPSR) is a set of rules that requires consumer products to be safe and our obligations to ensure this.*

*If you have any concerns about our products, you can contact us on ProductSafety@springernature.com*

In case Publisher is established outside the EU, the EU authorized representative is:

Springer Nature Customer Service Center GmbH
Europaplatz 3
69115 Heidelberg, Germany

**Batch number: 10620141**

Printed by Printforce, the Netherlands